Thank You
with a smile

**A personal battle with
mouth cancer**

Thank You
with a smile

A personal battle with mouth cancer

Christine Dunningham

*To my dear husband, Alan
who was with me every step of the way.*

Order this book online at www.trafford.com/08-0176
or email orders@trafford.com

Most Trafford titles are also available at major online book retailers.

Note for Librarians: A cataloguing record for this book is available from Library and Archives Canada at www.collectionscanada.ca/amicus/index-e.html

Design and typesetting by Matthew and Sandra Taylor
for *Start Design*

Photography by Alan & Jonathan Dunningham and Matt Taylor

Printed in Victoria, BC, Canada.

ISBN: 978-1-4251-7080-6

We at Trafford believe that it is the responsibility of us all, as both individuals and corporations, to make choices that are environmentally and socially sound. You, in turn, are supporting this responsible conduct each time you purchase a Trafford book, or make use of our publishing services. To find out how you are helping, please visit www.trafford.com/responsiblepublishing.html

Our mission is to efficiently provide the world's finest, most comprehensive book publishing service, enabling every author to experience success. To find out how to publish your book, your way, and have it available worldwide, visit us online at www.trafford.com/10510

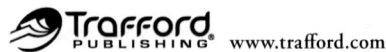

Trafford PUBLISHING® www.trafford.com

North America & international
toll-free: 1 888 232 4444 (USA & Canada)
phone: 250 383 6864 ♦ fax: 250 383 6804 ♦ email: info@trafford.com

The United Kingdom & Europe
phone: +44 (0)1865 487 395 ♦ local rate: 0845 230 9601
facsimile: +44 (0)1865 481 507 ♦ email: info.uk@trafford.com

10 9 8 7 6 5 4 3

Contents

Acknowledgements

A huge thank you to all the people who have been on this journey with me. You have accompanied and encouraged, given overwhelming prayer support and like Alan, been with me every step of the way. My thanks include all the members of the medical teams whose dedication and skill have given me confidence to carry on. I'm glad I'm not likely to have to write an Oscar speech as there are so many people that should be named within these pages that there wouldn't be room for the story! Everyone of you has been such a blessing to me and I thank God for your love and friendship, even those who have 'bullied' me into writing my story! The words "You should write a book" terrified me a year ago but by the grace of God and the persistence of my beloved husband, my family, and all of you, I've done it!

Thank you also to those of you who have given practical help in preparing this story ready for publication: Anne Warren, Diane Morrison, Stephen Rand and my husband, Alan.

Thank you to *CWR* for their permission to quote from the September/October 2006 issue of *Every Day with Jesus*.

Bible quotations are taken from the *New International Version* unless otherwise stated.

Foreword

It always seems to happen to somebody else. This time, that 'somebody else' was Christine Dunningham. I knew Christine as the wife of Alan, a colleague for many years at Tearfund. That was where I heard that she had cancer. Once again it had happened to 'somebody else.'

I did the usual things – told Alan how sorry I was. I kept in touch with the news as he passed it on to a circle of friends, many of them praying friends. I confess I didn't join those at Tearfund who met to pray for Christine; I was always too busy. It had happened to 'somebody else.'

For Alan, of course, it wasn't somebody else. It was the person he loved, the one he cared about the most. One of the privileges of reading this book is discovering how much someone can rise to the challenge when they are motivated by love that is then expressed in genuine selflessness and caring concern.

In one sense I am not surprised. I saw many of these positive qualities in the relationships Alan had at work. But what an encouragement to know that when put to the test, those qualities do not crumble, they do not only survive, but they are demonstrated even more profoundly. Christine writes about Alan with such appreciation: it is a testimony to marriage at its best, and a delight to read.

For Christine, this was not happening to somebody else; it was happening to her. I suspect I am not alone in occasionally wondering how I would react if it happened to me. Cancer has come close: both my parents died of it. Even so, my guess is none of us know how we will react until it does happen to us.

So some will be reading this book because they have been through a similar experience; others may be facing the start of the battle; some will be no more than onlookers.

But reading the story of Christine's rollercoaster ride with the big 'C' cannot fail to leave any reader unmoved. It reveals her own remarkable courage and perseverance; her dogged refusal to give up; her determination not to be beaten.

What's more, it reveals the vital importance of support from friends and family, the difference human relationships make to life. The older I get, the more I recognise the importance of investment in these relationships – Christine underlines that so clearly in these pages.

So all human life is here. Not only husband and wife; not only friends and family; not only dedicated and skilled nurses and doctors, surgeons and therapists: one other person is here as well. The sustaining love and care of God is not only expressed in and through all the people involved; Christine knows it herself, the result of the relationship with God through Jesus she has built over many years of faithfully sharing her life – good times and bad – with him.

For God, bad things never happen to somebody else; they happen to people he made in his image, people he loves, people he cares about, people he reaches out to as they reach for him.

For all these reasons, Christine, your book was worth writing. For all these reasons it is worth reading. And my prayer is that, above all, it will be a blessing to 'somebody else.'

Stephen Rand
Co Chair
Jubilee Debt Campaign

Introduction

"*There* is no easy way to tell you this, but you have a cancer called squamous cell carcinoma of the oral cavity."

Alan and I sat there in the consultant's office, stunned. You never think this is going to happen to you; it always happens to someone else. The night before, I had been at a Christmas party, little realising that the following day my life would change forever.

For eight years I had been treated and kept under surveillance at my local Ashford Hospital (Middlesex) for a condition of the gums called Lichen Planus. As it was becoming more painful and uncomfortable I had asked if I could have a second opinion and an appointment was arranged for me at Guy's Hospital, where I saw a very kind and caring consultant, Ms Pepe Shirlaw, Clinical Director for Dental Services and Consultant in Oral Medicine. On seeing the condition of my mouth she said, "I hope it is not what I think it is. I haven't seen this condition more than two or three times in the past five to ten years."

She stayed with me all afternoon, even though she was meant to be lecturing elsewhere, and arranged for me to have various tests and three biopsies. When the results were in she would contact Ashford hospital. The waiting period was difficult because, although cancer hadn't been mentioned, I suppose it was always at the back of our minds.

A few days later the telephone rang and I found myself speaking to Mr Creedon, Specialist in Oral Surgery at Ashford Hospital. By coincidence he was also looking after my mother who had been taken there the previous Sunday with a burst abscess in her jaw and had just had an operation on her mouth. He asked me if I was coming in to see her and I told him I was planning to visit that afternoon. When he asked if I could come in at twelve noon to see him, I assumed that he wanted to talk about my mother's condition; it just didn't occur to me that it was my situation he wanted to discuss.

I rang Alan at work, to tell him and he asked if I wanted him to come with me. I said no, because I was sure it had nothing to do with me, but a few minutes later he rang back to say he wanted to be there and would meet me in the car park. This can only be divine intervention in view of the devastating news I was about to receive.

I suppose in a way we were prepared for the diagnosis but not until it was confirmed did we think it actually could be cancer. I'd had a previous biopsy taken at Ashford only a few weeks before those done at Guy's, and it had come back clear, but a growth such as mine can turn cancerous overnight, and Mr Creedon wanted to tell me face to face and not over the telephone.

The first question I asked was, "Am I going to die?" Apparently this is often the first question people ask when told they have cancer. Mr Creedon said no, but indicated that I had a long haul ahead of me. First there had to be a lot of preliminary tests to go through – blood tests, scans, x-rays, photographs etc – which he would set up for me immediately. He told me that I would have to go to Kingston Hospital to meet as many of the team as possible who would be involved in the operation and possible radiotherapy. This appointment would be organised straight away; it was vital that my operation took place without delay, as this type of cancer escalates at a fast rate.

A nurse, Val, was in the room when the news was broken to me, and was to be with me during many of my future appointments. She fetched me a mug of tea while I tried to assimilate all this. Knowing that everything associated with a cancerous condition is 'bad news' and facing an unknown future left me feeling very scared. Alan immediately said, "I will be with you every step of the way." This meant so much to me – then and ever since. He has always been at all my appointments, always at my side helping, nursing, listening and being the most wonderful encourager. I know I am blessed to have such a faithful and caring husband.

Chapter One
Before My Life Turned Upside Down

*I*was born in May 1939 in Dringhouses, York, three years after my brother David, and just before the outbreak of the Second World War. My father, The Rev Kenneth Hawkins, moved to take up the position of Vicar of St Barnabas Church, which nestles in between York Station and the River Ouse. The river was so near that our garden was often flooded during the winter. York Station was bombed in 1942 and the vicarage had all the windows blown in; my mother saved me moments beforehand from my cot, which was a miracle in itself.

As a result of this my father decided to move to the South of England to take up the living at St Lawrence Church, Bovingdon, in Hertfordshire. It was here that my brother, Stephen, was born. It was on his second birthday that a severe thunderstorm hit Bovingdon early one Sunday evening while my father was taking the service. He was duly inspired as he preached on the 'Second Coming of Our Lord', challenging the congregation with the question, "Are you ready to face the Lord if called home tonight?" After the service he organised hymn singing until the torrential rain stopped. The churchyard was flooded and, as his Austin 7 was the only car small enough to go through the lych-gate, he waded through the water to bring it down to the main entrance. He took every member of the congregation home but then feeling ill, called at the doctor's house where he collapsed and died in his arms. He was just 35 years old. Daddy dying was quite a major event – a clergyman dying in situ in such circumstances hit all the national papers. My family had two hundred letters of sympathy from very prominent people, including archbishops.

My mother was left with three children to support plus her father-in-law who had recently come to live with us. My grandfather bought a house for us all and we moved to Watford. The Clergy Orphans' Corporation said they would educate my brothers and myself and so we were sent as boarders to St Edmund's, Canterbury and St Margaret's, Bushey respectively. It was very sad for my mother to have to part with her children to boarding school. I was only eight years old when I started at St Margaret's. I found boarding very difficult and cannot say that I look back on my school days with any particular joy; the only bright point was playing in the lacrosse team during my final year. It was hard too, as I only saw my mother once a fortnight on a Saturday afternoon between twelve noon and six o'clock. She caught a bus from our home on the Cassiobury Park Estate into Watford and then another bus taking her to Bushey and walked from there to my school. As the reverse journey took ages, I hardly spent any time at home, needing to return to St Margaret's by six o'clock in time for chapel. My mother made this journey every fortnight for eight years

I cannot pinpoint an actual day when I accepted Jesus Christ as my Saviour. I grew up in a Christian family and was educated in a Christian school, so Christianity was a part of my life. During the 1950s, Dr Billy Graham conducted crusades at both Wembley Arena and Harringay Stadium. My mother took me to quite a few of these meetings and on one occasion my school also took a party of girls to hear him. Listening to Dr Billy Graham had a great impact on my life as he explained the gospel so simply. I suddenly realised that I had to make a decision for myself to follow Jesus Christ and this I did in the quietude of my bedroom. Thus started my spiritual journey which has grown and matured over the years.

After leaving school at the age of sixteen, I trained in

shorthand and typing and gained my College Diploma, then I worked as a shorthand typist, and in due course graduated to being a secretary. My first job was at Rolls Royce in London although I never got to sit in one of their cars! The job that I enjoyed most was working for the Secretary for Training at the National Association of Boys' Clubs, London. It was there that I first heard about Cliff Richard, (now Sir Cliff Richard, of course) as he was discovered in the Cheshunt Boys' Club. He became a committed Christian and like many women of my age I have followed his career ever since.

In 1956 I met Alan at a local school dance when we were both 16 years old: he had taken another girl and I had gone with another boy but by the end of the evening it was a different story and we have stayed together ever since!

In the 1950s it was not thought proper that a boy and a girl should go on holiday without a chaperone, so 4 years later, Alan and I went for a holiday to my Godmother who lived in East Bergholt, Suffolk. This was a very beautiful part of England being 'Constable Country' and had special significance for me as I had slept in Willy Lott's Cottage (which was featured in John Constable's painting "The Hay Wain") while on a biology course at Flatford Mill. During the week we managed to escape our chaperone and Alan took me to the banks of the River Stour not far from Flatford Mill and asked me to marry him. I had longed for this day and was very excited when he presented me with a beautiful engagement ring.

Sadly, Alan's parents were not so happy, as they thought we were far too young to contemplate marriage and, as Alan hadn't 'played the field', they felt he couldn't possibly know if I was the 'right' one. One year later though, in 1961, we married at St Luke's Church, Watford and moved to our first home in Lee Green, London. Years later Alan's parents did say that we had obviously had a very happy marriage and that they had been proved wrong which was rather nice of them.

I know that both of us being strong Christians has played a big part in bonding us together to cope with whatever has been thrown at us. Marriage is like a rope. It can either have two strands or three. If the rope is made of two strands then it can easily be broken, but if it has three strands, then it is not so easily broken. We made God the Head of our marriage, so we had a cord of three strands – God, Alan and I – and this has held us together ever since. This idea comes from the Bible and is quoted in Ecclesiastes Ch 4 v 12.

On our honeymoon I slipped and fell down a cliff! This was to be the start of back problems that have plagued me for most of my life. I tried all sorts of treatments including many different and varied injections, to no avail and, eventually, I was told that I had a condition called Arachnoiditis (sounds like, but has no connection with spiders!) which we had never heard of. Then one consultant suggested, "Go to the gym and work through your pain" whatever that meant! So I presented myself at the gym and it was there I was introduced to Maurice, who is an osteopath. He was interested in my story and immediately was willing to 'have a go' and see if he could help. In 1994 he started treating me and little by little I got better. I shall always be grateful for his perseverance and encouragement over the years, which has enabled me to live a more normal life. I call him 'my miracle man' and I can hear many people who I have referred to him say, "hear, hear!"

We have four wonderful children, Andrew, Jonathan, Peter and Mary, who are all now happily married, and we have been blessed with four beautiful grandchildren, Emily, Annabel, Jack and Daisy, who give us a great deal of pleasure. During the first part of our married life we moved seven times while Alan was working in the sports trade until we eventually settled in Shepperton, Middlesex, after a change of career when Alan joined Tearfund (a Christian Third World Relief and Development Agency) as General Manager of their trading company, Tearcraft.

This was to be very interesting and rewarding work that helped us to make friends worldwide. These people have enriched our lives and given us tremendous prayer support during difficult times.

Our family regularly attend All Saints' Church, Laleham, and we are involved in many activities within the church family. We used to enjoy camping and attended many Christian holiday camps around the country.

In 2000, our daughter, Mary, asked me to make her wedding cake, and this led me into the hobby of sugar craft, which I now really enjoy. Gena, the mother of one of her bridesmaids, was a teacher of sugar craft and had been intending to make her cake, but she was going to Australia at the time of the wedding. Gena spent a whole day with me explaining the mechanics of how to go about it and then left me to get on with it – a challenge I nervously took up! Although we didn't realise at the time, this was to be the start of a very special friendship.

Chapter Two
Love Outpoured

One of the hardest things I had to do after hearing the shocking and sad news that I had cancer was to visit my mother. I didn't want her to know my prognosis because she was ninety-seven years old and I was afraid of how it might affect her. So I braced myself and put on a smile, while inside, all I wanted to do was cry, and I tried to cheer her up when all I wanted was for my mother to cheer me up. From then onwards, for the next week or so, I would visit my mother daily, putting on a brave face in the ward while talking to the doctor or nurse, and then outside being instructed by the same people to go for the next test in preparation for the big team visit at Kingston. This was scheduled for Christmas Eve 2003 and in the meantime I was advised to make a list of all my questions – we certainly had a lot to ask!

When we got home after my diagnosis, we had barely got our coats off when there was a knock at the door and there stood Joan (a friend from our church). She was going to put a card of encouragement about something totally different through the letter box, but felt she ought to knock. This again was divine intervention. After we had shared our awful news, she was the first person to pray for us as we started on our long journey through a very dark tunnel. I always refer to 'we' because the one who is nearest and dearest, my beloved husband, Alan, had to bear the emotional strain. News travels quite fast in our church and later that afternoon our Vicar's wife, Meg, arrived bearing a beautiful bouquet of yellow roses. This meant so much to us and was the beginning of many beautiful flowers which were to flood into our home during the coming months.

That evening Alan telephoned our three boys to let them know our devastating news, but our daughter, Mary, was travelling the world for a year with her husband, Lee. Alan was unable to contact her and had to wait until she telephoned us on the 19th December to tell her the news, when she immediately asked if she should come home. This was a question we put to our Consultant when we met him in Kingston, but he said, "no" as the operation itself was not life-threatening. Mary telephoned on Christmas Day to find out the result of the CT scan and the other tests and was relieved to hear that the cancer had not spread. It was very hard for her to be so far away during this traumatic family time. One of the good things though was that, from January to May, Mary worked at a hospital in Auckland as a Speech Therapist and therefore it was easier for her to keep in touch through e-mails.

Recently I asked my children how they each felt after we had told them that I had been diagnosed with cancer, this is what they told me:

Andrew:
- Shock and disbelief – this was the type of thing that happened to other people, in other families – not to my Mum, to my family.
- Anxiety about Mum's future – just how bad was the cancer? Possibility of really unpleasant treatment without a good result – as later happened to Ray.
- Huge sympathy for Mum – particularly distressing for a woman to undergo surgery that will disfigure her face; also, Mum loves to talk! So huge sympathy that her voice might be affected.
- Sympathy for Mum and Dad – with Dad approaching retirement; would their retirement be very different from

the one that they had worked hard for and dreamed of?

- Sense of unfairness – whilst acknowledging that no cancer is fair – but she had not smoked or drank – it just seemed so unfair.

- Sympathy for Grandy* – in her late 90s and frail, to see her only daughter so ill and – a practical point – unable to visit – desire to "protect" Grandy and to be in more regular contact with her.

- Sense of beginning of role reversal – need to protect and support my parents as they had done for the Grans for so long and for my siblings and I.

- Feeling of huge responsibility to provide as much practical help as possible – with a very busy life, this required prioritising. I spoke to our vicar and reduced my responsibilities at church; Liz stepped down as school governor. We explained to friends that supporting Mum and Dad was our priority for 2004 and asked for prayer support, but explained that we would be doing less socialising. We wanted to be able to visit frequently; I also felt it was very important to be with Dad whilst Mum was undergoing surgery.

- Bowled over by the support and practical help, eg offers of help looking after the children by many friends. Really kind and thoughtful responses, but in a way this made Mum's situation more real. People were very kind and continue to ask after Mum's health three years later.

- Sense of the ground beneath my feet shifting. Mum had always been there; now the future seemed a lot less clear.

- Need to pray for Mum's recovery and strength for Dad.

- Proud of my children, aged five, eight and ten, who all accepted that Grandma would need lots of love, support and visits, even if this meant missing things that they would have liked to have done, eg birthday parties.

- Overwhelmingly, I felt that I wanted to be a faithful, loving son – this awful situation was not about me, it was about my Mum and Dad and I wanted to be a good son.

*(*Grandy* was the name Andrew gave to my mother at a very early age and it just stuck)

Jonathan:
- Shock ... Don't want to loose my mummy yet. Let's pray that it's not God's time to take Mum home and that, if it is, He'll change His mind!
- Let's pray that mum is strong enough to get through this and that she wants to.

Peter:
Obviously, I was completely gutted, to think that my Mummy could have the 'dreaded one' was unimaginable ... others get this don't they? Not in my family ... surely? This news was sudden and caught us completely unaware. Why Mum? What has she ever done wrong to deserve this? She doesn't smoke, drink or eat bad foods... why? This surely can't be true, what about all the others who abuse themselves and are still healthy people? Why does this always happen to the good people, this just isn't fair, but then again life generally isn't, is it?

Mary:
I remember feeling totally heartbroken and useless and hopeless that I couldn't do anything. Also guilt ridden that I could get on a plane and come home, and yet I didn't. I don't think I'll ever get over that and I feel like crying now. I felt pulled between you and Lee (her husband), and I know Lee would have supported me whatever, and I know for sure that I was led by what your consultant told you that your life wasn't immediately in danger but ... I felt

hollow inside and to be honest I was being quite selfish in my thoughts, thinking things like, you may not see my first child and how could I ever carry on without my mum … We found out in a phone box in Christchurch (New Zealand) and Lee and I walked around for hours until Lee said I should eat something but I really found it difficult to eat. We talked for hours and met up with Rik and Jon (our travelling companions while in New Zealand) and Lee told them so they left us alone for the evening. I didn't sleep at all that night … oh dear the tears have come …

Gena's husband, Ray, was diagnosed with cancer of the mouth at Ashford Hospital, in November 2003, a month before I received the same diagnosis. Ray's operation was on the 16th December at St George's hospital, London, and it was just after this that I telephoned Gena to find out how Ray was and to break the news to her that I too had just been told I had cancer of the mouth. There was a long silence while Gena tried to take this in. She could hardly believe it as we were both under the same consultant and, although I had a different type of cancer, I would be going through similar procedures.

After the dust had settled somewhat, we pursued many different avenues that might be helpful in supporting me through the forthcoming weeks. A friend gave me a list of different ideas, one of which was to get in touch with the Bristol Cancer Help Centre. We received from them a self-help pack that included a video, all of which we found very helpful and informative. However, we decided not to proceed with going on their course because time was short and it was going to be difficult to fit it in before my operation. Also it was very expensive and over a hundred miles away.

We were given the name of an organisation called *Breath Ministries*, which is the umbrella name that Christian Alternative

Thank You - with a smile

ERRATA
Page 12 – 1 John 4 v 8 should read
Jeremiah 29 v 11
Page 13 – Isaiah 46 v 3 & 4 should read
Ephesians 3 v 20 & 21

Therapies work under. Alan rang them up and was given the name of a homeopath who lived locally. We decided to go and have a talk with her before committing ourselves, as I wanted to be sure that I would be comfortable with her helping me alongside all my doctors. I also needed to know if my consultant, would be happy for me to be supported in this way – he was. We visited Cathy and she told us all about her approach to my condition and how we would work together not only to prepare me for the operation but also to help me through the operation period and into the future. Alan questioned her in depth and wanted to know all there was to know about homeopathy. We immediately took to her and felt that homeopathy could play an important part in the preparation and recovery period but I would have to play my part. She explained that the type of food I eat is very important and she wanted me to buy organic food wherever possible to eliminate certain chemicals passing into my body. She put me on a special regime, which I found very difficult to keep to because I had not been treated by homeopathy before, but I was determined to persevere. Immediately after the operation I carried on with my treatment, part of which included giving me remedies to strengthen my bones in the hope that in the future, I might be able to have implants in my jaw to hold new teeth. She also recommended that I took various vitamin supplements to build up my immune system. Cathy has been a wonderful help, support and encourager and she still keeps an eye on me!

A few weeks before discovering I had cancer, friends of ours in New Zealand, Alan and Lesley, e-mailed us about a book called *The Purpose Driven Life* by Rick Warren, which had spoken to their hearts. A couple of days after my diagnosis I was reading this book and the following caught my attention:

"I know what I am planning for you … 'I have good plans for you, not plans to hurt you. I will give you hope and a good future'" 1 John 4 v 8.

The book said that, however impossible the situation might seem,

"*God ... is able to do far more than we would ever dare to ask or even dream of – infinitely beyond our highest prayers, desires, thoughts, or hopes*" Isaiah 46 v 3–4

On the same day, the Lord woke Alan early in the morning with two verses of assurance:

"*Trust in the Lord with all your heart and lean not on your own understanding: in all your ways acknowledge Him, and He will make your paths straight*" Proverbs 3 v 5 and 6

He typed these verses out in large letters and stuck them on our bedroom mirror.

After two days of utter despair, many tears and sleepless nights interspersed with gallons of tea, we knew that the only way forward was to commit our situation into God's hands and trust Him for the future. I tried to stay positive and not let Satan take over but I must confess there were many times when I kept asking the question, "Why?" Alan was so strong and courageous, he would sit me down, let me talk endlessly and never complained.

On Christmas Eve we presented ourselves at Kingston Hospital to meet some of the team who would be involved with my treatment over the next months. One of these was Mr Malcolm Bailey (Consultant Oral and Maxillofacial Surgeon) who although based at Ashford, I had not yet had the pleasure of meeting. He turned out to be very highly respected in his field and I was very happy to trust myself to his care. It also transpired that he was a Christian, which was an added joy and assurance to Alan and me. At this meeting we also met the lady who was to be my oncologist, Dr Sarah Partridge (Consultant in Clinical Oncology). I think everyone was quite interested in my condition because it was so rare. I was told that the operation would be at St George's Hospital, Tooting, London, and would last about twelve hours.

The result of my CT scan showed that there was no further spread of cancer which was a great relief. Mr Bailey told us that he would try and get the team together as quickly as possible and hoped he may be able to operate on either the 13th or 20th January, 2004. Owing to the Christmas holiday period it was not possible to put a large team together by the earlier date and eventually I was informed that, providing there was a bed available, the operation would take place on the 20th January 2004.

During this waiting period our family and friends were so loving and kind, reaching out to us in many different ways. We had flowers, cards, e-mails, letters, and offers of help even before I had got to hospital. It was this outpouring of love towards us that helped to get us through those difficult weeks. I cannot emphasise enough the importance of people as they touched our lives.

Gena and Ray were also a tremendous support to us at this time. The day after Ray came out of hospital he wrote me a long e-mail giving me some idea of what might happen to me, giving me as much preparation as possible, as I was to follow him into the same ward. One of the very practical things he said was: "In case you have a tracheotomy, make sure to take a notebook and pencil with you so that you can convey to the nurses what it is you want of them – very frustrating without. Make sure the pencil/pen is attached to the pad so it can't get lost, and keep the notebook handy." As I found out later, this was a very sound piece of advice and one I was very thankful for. When I look back at how I felt when I came out of hospital, writing this e-mail was a very courageous and loving thing for Ray to do. He too had a strong Christian faith and was trying to help me as much as possible because he knew what I would be facing. I shall always be grateful for his forethought and care for me when he was suffering so much himself.

Gena sent me a poem, which had been sent to Ray as an encouragement and I quote it here:

Though I know not what awaits me
What the future has in store,
Yet I know that God is faithful
For I've proved Him oft before. (Anon)

Then a few days before I went into hospital, Gena came to see me, to give me encouragement and also brought a gift – a hand-held food blender. I looked at it and was very polite and thanked her profusely but inside I was thinking, "why would I need that?" Gena said I would need one after my stay in hospital and I looked at her in disbelief because I hadn't really taken in the fact that I wouldn't be able to eat normally. Of course, Gena understood my needs and was being very practical. I shall never be more thankful to her for her foresight in giving me this wonderful gift, which I still use most days. It is also my travelling companion.

At this time Alan worked in the fundraising team at *Tearfund*. They all agreed to stop work each morning for half an hour to pray for us both for one month. This was such a wonderful thing for them to do, and we are so grateful, not only for their love and support, but also to the whole of Tearfund for their prayers. Just before I started radiotherapy Alan's team presented us with a folder containing thoughts and verses which the Lord had given them during their prayer time together. One or two other people had also added a word of encouragement. This meant so much to us and is very precious.

Chapter Three
Black Thursday

My gums were very painful and my bottom teeth very wobbly and so I just longed for my operation to take place. I naively thought that once my teeth were taken out all would be well and I would be out of pain – well I was in for a very rude awakening! At long last I was summoned to St George's for further pre-op tests and preparation on 15th January 2004. We call it '*Black Thursday*'. A few days before this took place I was telephoned to say that an appointment had been made for 3 pm on my pre-op day to have a minor operation to insert a PEG *(Percutaneous Endoscopic Gastrostomy)* into my stomach. I had no idea what this meant but on further investigation found out that it was to feed me after the operation as I wouldn't be able to eat anything through my mouth.

We presented ourselves at St George's feeling that we were one step nearer the operation but with no idea what was in store. I would like to blot this day out of my memory.

First of all, we were introduced to the other Consultant Maxillofacial Surgeon, Mr Nicholas Hyde, who would be sharing the operation. He was delightful and immediately put us at ease. He told us that the cancer appeared to be more extensive than had been previously thought and was growing fast! It extended down into the jaw, which meant that a section of jaw would have to be removed in addition to the teeth, gums and lymph glands. This bone would have to be replaced by some bone, artery, veins and skin from the leg. It was then explained to us that I would have to go into hospital a day earlier so they could carry out a special test on my legs to find the best piece of bone to take for grafting into the jaw. They were not sure how much bone would be needed; if possible they would take bone from the left arm but they had to be ready for any eventuality. I then spent a long time with the *'two Jo's'*, a Dietician and a Speech and Language Therapist (hereafter referred to as SLT). They were delightful and ready to give us as much time as we needed. It was then that I was told I would have to have a tracheotomy. So not only was I to get food through a tube, I was also only going to be able to breathe through a tube! It was during this time that we were told that I might never be able to talk again or eat or drink again through my mouth. I had no idea what I would look like except that my lower lip would slant inwards as there would be no teeth to support it. In a nutshell I was given all the worst case scenarios to prepare me for what lay ahead.

I was then sent for further tests including x-rays, blood tests, ECG, and photographs before reporting to the department to have my PEG fitted. Again, I had no idea what to expect and by this time I was quite depressed. When I reached the relevant department Alan had to leave me and I was given a bed to lie on while I waited. I was feeling very down and alone, when a student nurse called Sue was suddenly standing by me and started talking to me to try and ease my nerves. She will never know what a comfort she was to me, as she kept me chatting while I waited my turn and she promised to stay with me throughout the procedure. As a student nurse, she was spending time on that unit observing the fitting of PEGs. She seemed very interested in my condition and asked me if she could follow my whole treatment through, as this would help her with learning and understanding a patient's journey. Sue got permission from Mr Bailey to observe my operation.

When I came to (having been heavily sedated while the PEG was fitted), I found I had a long tube inserted in my stomach and I was instructed how to keep this clean. I was in quite a bit of pain and told not to eat anything that night. The pain didn't last more than a day or two but having a tube sticking out of my tummy was a bit of a nuisance! This, in due course, was linked up to special liquid food bags and a pump that fed me, usually during the night! The downside to this was that I had to sit up all night and it was to be about six months before I would be able to lie down and sleep naturally.

When Alan and I were eventually able to leave the hospital we both knew that our lives would be very different in the future, but I still didn't really understand what lay ahead for me. I did feel frightened and scared despite the sure knowledge that God was with me. I only had two days before I had to report back to the hospital – there was a lot to do.

Having said goodbye to all my friends at our church, it was time to get myself organised. It wasn't only the things to take into hospital that I had to get ready, I also needed to leave our home in order so that Alan had as little to do as possible. I asked my friends at church to "look after my Alan"; I was concerned about him, as I knew he had to cope with the emotional strain, visiting, working, looking after the home and, not least, cooking for himself. He is no cook and has always boycotted the kitchen! Our church fellowship was a tower of strength to us both, for which we shall always be so grateful and thankful.

Elizabeth, married to our eldest son Andrew, wrote me many helpful letters and cards and, being a nurse, sent a very practical one before I went into hospital advising me as to the best things to take. Andrew telephoned his father a few days before my operation and asked him what he was going to do while I was in the operating theatre. Alan said he didn't know and hadn't even thought about it. Andrew then asked him if he would like him to come and be with him. This was such a loving thought and I encouraged Alan to say yes. A few days later Alan told Andrew that it would be good to have him by his side.

Jonathan and Anne, came to see us the day before I went into

St George's and brought me a very attractive 'goodie bag' full of tiny gifts. Anne said she was sure Mary, our daughter, would have done this but in her absence wanted to be her substitute. This was so thoughtful and, of course, brought tears to my eyes.

Peter, our youngest son who lived locally, wanted to cook us a meal so it was arranged for the Sunday of my admittance. In quite an emotional state, I felt it would be too hard going to church again so we asked our vicar, Peter, if he would kindly bring communion to our home. This he gladly did and then Alan and I went to our Peter's home where Andrew, Elisabeth and our three grandchildren, Emily, Annabel and Jack joined us, having travelled up from Taunton in Somerset. Peter laid on the most amazing roast dinner but he made for me something entirely different and special. I was so touched, as even then I had difficulty in eating because my teeth were so wobbly and painful. I think we were all feeling emotional because none of us knew what the outcome of the operation would be. The children were so quiet I wondered if they had been primed by their parents to be extra especially good! After lunch we went into the garden with the camera and took a few pictures. I had got together a few family photos, which I often looked at while in hospital.

I mentioned earlier how helpful Alan and I had found *The Purpose Driven Life* by Rick Warren so we decided to give a copy to each of our four children and their families. We asked Mary and Lee to buy a copy in New Zealand (which, of course, we would pay for) so that in some way we were all linked together. This they did and amazingly found that the church they were attending was following a course of Bible studies based on this book!

And so the time had come to say goodbye to our family and make the journey to St George's Hospital. I found this very hard; there were hugs all round and, as Alan drove away, the tears began to fall. There was certainly no backing out, as I knew that the only way to save my life was to go through with this big operation.

Chapter Four
Signing My Life Away

I had been asked to present myself at Dalby Ward, Lanesborough Wing, St George's Hospital, at 4 pm on Sunday 18th January 2004. My heart was pounding as we reached the ward where I was told to wait until a nurse was free to come and admit me. At that moment I had a feeling of not belonging anywhere – being in a sort of limbo state – and I longed to be shown to my bed and start to get myself sorted out. Until I got to know the procedures and some of the nurses, it all seemed very strange but after a while I became acclimatised. I suppose it was a bit like moving house and having to get to know the new district. It was hard saying goodbye to Alan but, of course, I knew he would be back again the next day after I had had the test on my legs.

The test showed that I had three arteries in my left leg but only two in my right leg! This meant that if bone and an artery had to be taken from a leg then it would have to be from the left one. I certainly didn't want this to happen because that would weaken the leg and, having had about six operations on my left foot, broken the left ankle and pulled all the ligaments in that leg in a skiing accident many years before, I felt my right leg would have been the better option! We would have to wait on that decision until the operation.

That same evening Alan was with me when the House Surgeon came to explain to me all about what they might and might not do at the operation and that he had to get my consent. One thing that hadn't been mentioned before was the possibility that I might have to have a 'split lip', but in the event they were able to cut round my neck to gain access to the inside of my mouth. He also told me that I had to take off any rings including my wedding ring. I told him that I had never removed it since Alan had put it on my finger over forty-two years ago – I was just told that if I didn't remove the ring then there would be no operation!

I was then given what seemed like endless forms to sign and it really felt as if I was signing my life away. As we were engaged in this exercise the evening meal came round. I had been really looking forward to a last meal but by the time I had completed all the formalities, the trolley had gone and I had been left some cold cottage pie! I shall never forget my frustration and that dreadful last meal.

So the last thing Alan did for me that evening was to get my ring off using a lot of soap! It may seem something quite small to some people, but to me it was another blow. Actually, when the swelling eventually went down in my hand, I had to have my ring made smaller because I had lost a lot of weight.

After Alan had left me, promising to be back with Andrew at 7 am the next morning, as we were not sure at what time I would be taken to theatre, I had a lovely chat with the young lady in the bed opposite and later we corresponded for quite a while by e-mail. I am so glad that e-mails have been invented because it makes it so much quicker and easier to keep in touch with people.

Alan decided that, as so many people were asking after me it would probably be helpful all round if he wrote an 'update' at intervals to keep our friends informed of how things were going. He sent out over a hundred e-mails all over the world and a further twenty by post. We knew the power of prayer and we also knew that if we wanted people to pray constructively, then keeping them informed of my progress would be helpful. Actually, the updates have been a very useful tool in remembering how things evolved and when I came to write this book, they helped to refresh my memory.

Of course, the breakfast trolley passed me by on the day I don't remember much about! It was wonderful to see Alan and Andrew at 7 am as we then had quite a wait because if a bed did not become available in the Intensive Care Unit, I would not be able to have my operation that day. I also had a visit from Sue, my lovely student nurse, who was with me when I had my PEG fitted and had received permission from Mr Bailey to be at my operation. It was not until 9 am that we got the message that the operation could go ahead and then it was all systems go and, in no time at all, I was on my way with Alan to theatre where I would be for the next fourteen hours. Sue met us before we reached the anaesthetic suite with a welcoming smile. When I asked her what she remembered about this time she told me:

"This point really sticks in my mind because you were making Alan laugh and being very brave. He had tears in his eyes which made me get tears in mine and bless him, when it was time for me and you to go into the room, he kissed you and gave me a hug and a kiss on the cheek too! I was very touched at how supportive he had been every time I had seen you two together and how obvious it was that he truly, truly loved you. I held your hand lots (both before, for the PEG, and during the time they put you to sleep) and then I stayed with you in the operating theatre for over eleven hours I think – I know I was knackered anyhow!! I remember not getting home till well after midnight. I then came and visited you on Dalby Ward a few times which was lovely, 'cos I got hugs from you, met more of your relatives and although you couldn't speak, your eyes said lots!"

A couple of years later we were delighted to hear from Sue that she had graduated with a distinction and had also won the Southwest London Strategic Health Authority award for the best overall performance. We were absolutely overjoyed for her, but not at all surprised because her dedication to the nursing profession really shone through.

We had heard that Mr Bailey was a Christian through a friend at our church, so Alan wrote him a note before the operation just to let him know that many people would be praying for him and the whole team. One of our friends, Mavis, organised for our church, All Saints', Laleham, to be open from 10 am to 4 pm specifically for prayer for me and my medical team knowing that it was going to be a very long operation. Many people came throughout the day and I feel very humbled, grateful and thankful to God for so many special people who took time out to pray.

After Alan had left me, he and Andrew went straight down to the hospital chapel to pray. Even there, the Lord was to be an encouragement to them as Andrew recognised the Chaplain as a minister he knew from Taunton. Sadly, with repairs going on just outside the chapel, it was almost impossible to meditate and pray there so they left for home. They told me that they then went to our church in Laleham and spent some time in prayer. After that, both being golfers, they decided to go to the local driving range and hit about a hundred golf balls for all they were worth! They imagined the indentations on the balls were cancer cells and it was their way of trying to get rid of them! Alan said, "It was wonderful how at various points during the day, things 'happened' that confirmed God's presence with us and we felt greatly supported although we also experienced some darker moments."

In the evening they enjoyed a lovely meal by kind invitation of Mavis and Bruce who had organised the opening of the church to support our family in prayer. They told Alan about the time their son Christopher was in hospital having a major heart operation and wanted to be well enough to perform in a concert two weeks later, so they took photos to show how he had progressed. Alan thought this was a lovely idea so he decided that, when he came to see me the next day, he would come armed with a camera. As a result we now have an amazing pictorial record of what I went through and as I look at them now four years later, I can hardly believe it is the same person!

Later that evening Mr Bailey himself telephoned Alan to say that the operation had gone very smoothly, they were close to finishing, and that I would soon be in the Intensive Care Unit. This was wonderfully reassuring for Alan to know, and Mr Bailey also confirmed that they had not had to use any bone from my leg. Alan told me that he and Andrew had slept much better that night having given thanks to Almighty God for His great love for me. It was such a relief for Alan to know that all had gone well and, in fact, the operation had lasted for fourteen hours.

The next time I was aware of anything was when I regained consciousness in the Intensive Care Unit the next day, but I don't really remember much until Alan and Andrew came to visit me later that day. I remember being in this amazingly quiet place with many complicated machines all round me. I couldn't move because I had so many tubes attached to my body and my left arm was being held in a vertical position. I had a silver necklace made up of many staples securing the wound round my neck and a lovely swollen face. It was like being in a vice. I couldn't speak because of the tracheotomy and I couldn't hear because I didn't have my hearing aids in – I couldn't even hear what my dedicated nurse said. When Alan arrived he realised what the problem was and got a nurse to fetch my hearing aids from my ward. Even then it was difficult to hear what was being said and, of course, I couldn't answer which was a great frustration. I had been warned that I wouldn't be able to speak but at that early stage I was not able to have my notebook and was much too weak even to hold a pencil let alone write with it. Of course, I was also unable to have anything to eat or drink so time passed very slowly indeed. It was to be many months before I even began to enjoy the cup of tea that many of us take so much for granted in our English way of life. There was not even a clock to tell me what time it was or how long I had been there. I was in my own personal hell, which was to continue for quite a while even when I was transferred to the High Dependency Ward. I think it will haunt me forever.

Of course, it was wonderful to see Alan and Andrew and they were a great encouragement to me but it was very hard to see them go not having been able to say anything to them. My dedicated nurse was very kind and she looked after me with such devotion. Before Alan went, he got my personal CD player and left me listening to a selection of Psalms with modern arrangements – a great favourite of mine. The only problem was that once the CD came to an end I couldn't indicate that it had finished in order for anyone to change it or at least put it on again. I was completely helpless and wondered what the future held.

Later on that evening I was moved to the High Dependency Unit within the ICU, which was darker with just a few dim lights on, and I passed a very long night wondering when morning would ever come. How I longed just to be able to move a little, but that was quite impossible.

The next time Alan saw me, I was back in my own ward but this time in the High Dependency Unit. I was still attached to many tubes and wires but at least I could watch the comings and goings of the hospital. I will never forget the heat in that ward and Alan had to get out all my summer nighties even though it was in the middle of winter! Alan told me that, as he and Andrew had been so encouraged by my condition, Andrew had decided to head back to Taunton, his task of caring for, and encouraging his dad now completed.

When alone I faced a real problem if the communication bell fell off the bed or it was left out of reach. As I couldn't move or speak, this at times, proved an insurmountable problem! As soon as I was back on the ward I started trying to communicate by the use of my notebook and pen. My hand was so weak that my writing was hardly legible – when Jonathan and his wife, Anne, came with Alan at the weekend we had a lot of fun as they tried to make out what I had written! As I got stronger the writing became more understandable. This is the way I would talk to the consultants and doctors as they came to check on my progress; I would try and have the questions written down before they arrived.

The next great event was the arrival of the SLT. She had come to gauge my potential for speech with the use of a 'speech valve'. I was so nervous in case I had lost the ability to speak, but the signs were good. Sadly, I developed a lung infection that needed treatment and prevented use of the valve over the weekend. This was a great disappointment to me but I knew I would have to be patient. This was one of the main lessons I would have to learn over the next months and years of my life. Everything took a long time and nothing was instant!

The Physiotherapist arrived to give me breathing exercises because, when lying in bed, it is very easy to get a lung infection. So to help me get better and prevent it from happening again, I had to start being good and have a go at these exercises. I am not very fond of exercises but I did my best. On one evening round Mr Hyde noticed that my tracheotomy was half out and immediately began to make me cough. I have never coughed so much in my life and for half an hour it was continual and very painful. Mr Hyde said he had to do it as my life was in danger. My throat continued to be very irritable for the rest of the evening, but I realised how fortunate I was that he had noticed this real threat to my life.

Every day, and quite often twice a day, I had blood taken from my good arm and I began to wonder if they would drain me dry! Tony Hancock's sketch 'The Blood Donor' seemed suddenly to make a lot of sense! There was one particular haematologist who was very jovial and I nicknamed him 'the blood man'. He always had a smile, which helped to cheer me up.

By the time Alan came to visit on the Monday, my infection had almost gone and the SLT had fitted the speech valve. I greeted Alan with a deep, Dalek-like, sexy voice (his description!). It was such a relief and joy to know that I would be able to speak again on my own once the tracheotomy had been removed. As I'd had several of the wires and tubes taken away we were able to take a few steps around the ward and corridors to help me with mobility and breathing capacity.

One week after my operation my surgeon and doctors detached all remaining support equipment except the feeding tube in my stomach which would have to stay with me for many months to come. The great moment then arrived when my SLT approved the removal of my tracheotomy tube allowing me to breathe normally, but with considerable effort, through my nose and mouth. I was told always to remember to place my hand over the dressing covering the old tracheotomy hole whenever I spoke or coughed, to enable healing.

I was excited when I was told that the dressing on my arm was due to come off because they wanted to see if the graft had taken and then the stitches could come out. It was quite a horrible and gory sight to me but the surgeon was delighted with it! A nurse spent simply ages picking out all the tiny stitches. I then had to have my arm put into a plaster, which completely immobilised my elbow.

Not being able to sleep at night because of the intense heat, I decided that I would use the time to write to my daughter, Mary, in New Zealand. Of course I missed her but I also had this idea that if I could pour out my feelings and frustrations to her in this way it might help her to feel part of my life even though she was so far away. These letters, which helped Mary to feel more involved with my progress, form my next chapter.

Chapter Five

Letters to my daughter

I wrote to Mary while I was in hospital and often during the night when I couldn't sleep:

Friday 23rd January 2004

Dearest Mary,
*   I am OK but still in hell! You know what I mean. I understand what you went through.* (Mary had a big operation for Scoliosis in the National Hospital in London in 2000.) *I have a chest infection and fun and games last evening. X-rays etc in ward just like you. The trach is horrible but my SLT is lovely. Everyone is kind. I have been told that they are doing their part and I have to as well – I'm not sure what they mean. What do I have to do? I can see no end to this. I will try and fight for you all but it is hard. I miss you so much. I think of you and Lee also the boys and grandchildren and of course my beloved Alan. I am SO hot.*

*   Lots of love,*
*   Mummy*

Sunday 25th January 2004

Dearest Mary,

Every time they do something horrible to me I think how brave you were. We know what suffering is all about. When I think of you I think positive because you made it. They are pleased with my chest today. Better night. Catheter came off today now scared about asking for the loo! You understand that I know. Felt sick this morning in the pit of my tummy – PEG FOOD URGH! They gave me some Gaviscon. A lot of wires came off today and a lot of playing around with my neck and I think some stitches were taken out. I shall never complain about being cold again. It is like the tropics here and I sometimes feel faint with the heat. Everyone seems pleased with me and I think of the grandchildren a lot and their little lives ahead of them. Everyone must make the best time of what God has given them and I am glad you have taken the plunge to do what you always wanted to. Well done. Even if you are broke!

I asked one of my surgeons if he thought he had got all the cancer cells and he said they had sent the bone to the lab for testing in cross sections and the results would be in 2/3 weeks. If there are cells still there then that is where the radiotherapy comes in. So we pray on in hope. Everyone has been fantastic. The boys are looking after Dad, also our wonderful Church Family. The love of Jesus is very special to experience. Very anxious about loo and wish my catheter was still in. Didn't have to worry then! I just go with the flow. Your body is not your own anymore!! Some nurses are super and nothing is too much trouble. Haven't got anything simple to read. Got to be very simple, romantic etc and big print!

Went to sleep last night listening to Classical FM and drifted in and out of that all night. The sound on the TV is very low and no subtitles. Dad got me 'Home and Away' off the Internet but I think it was well advanced!

As you cannot be here I have to chat to you in this way!

Trisha's mother has died – so sad for them when I am like this as well. They say it all comes at once.

I think you're going to be a fisherman's widow as well as a surfer widow!! Fishing must be so boring.

I had better stop otherwise poor Dad will never get to bed!!

Felt very weepy when they had finished with me but better now I have had a chat with you. Dad, JJ and Anne will be here in about 2-3 hours. Seems ages to wait. Sitting up is not much fun especially when you cannot move around but I must for my chest – being positive! Trying!

> *Lots of love, hugs and kisses,*
> *Mummy*

PS I have just been to wee – yippee!
Still feel very sick
Exhausted and back to bed after 2 hours in chair

Monday 26th January 2004

Dearest Mary,

I hope my daily updates are helping you to feel involved with progress.

I had a lovely time with Dad, JJ and Anne yesterday – always sad to see them go but I did have a good night in spite of sitting up all night. I slept from 10 pm – 3 am – had a loo stop and enjoyed sitting on commode for a change of scene! Then slept till 7 am! Of course, breakfast passed me by.

The Docs came round about 8 am and gave their orders for the day but I didn't hear what they were saying. They do quite a lot of teaching. I think they are quite interested in my case.

I then had my bed bath and by now I have it taped and won't let them away without washing every bit and 'lotioning' me!!! They got me sitting out by 10 am – quite a record.

Then the dietician came. I seem to be being fed all the time. Lots of wind but no movement!

Then my lovely SLT came with the Senior Staff Nurse and Macmillan Nurse. The SLT fitted a voice box and suddenly I can talk!! I can also suck a bit of saliva and they had done something to the trach to give me more oxygen up in the mouth. I might get rid of the trach in a couple of days – here's hoping. It might not be too long before I can have a heavenly sip of water. I kept thinking of you as the SLT was helping me. She wears a long black skirt and I think would be very similar in her work to you. She is so kind and encouraging. When I say I can talk – it sounds funny and false but quite amazing. Dad will get a surprise this afternoon.

He is well looked after which is wonderful but he won't learn to cook! But it is lovely for him being with different people each evening.

I can get my lips together now but cannot get all the saliva away yet so dribble a lot. I have to keep practising swallowing. I'm trying to tell you all this, as you understand the mechanics.

A new young lad has come in during the night opposite me. Chews gum all the time, on the telephone, has his top off and is a bit like Jack the lad – big boots! They are all men in this ward.

They seem to need blood every day and sometimes twice. Soon I won't have any left!

Just watched 'Home and Away' for first time since coming in but cannot hear very well. Wish they could do sub-titles. Very thoughtless for people in hospital. I really will have to set the world to right!!

I keep thinking of you. Sounds as if you had a lovely weekend. So glad you have some Christians surrounding you.

The man in the next bed has just gone and at last the curtain has been pulled back and I can see the London landscape. A rather grey day.

Think this is all for now.
Keep smiling dear and lots of love to you and Lee,
Mummy

PS Great news just walked to loo for 1st time!

Tuesday 27th January 2004

Dearest Mary,
Well, here goes for the Update. I get Dad to read it so I don't have to try and tell him, so it serves two purposes!

Since I finished writing last lunchtime, I had a lovely time with Dad talking with my bionic voice. Dad says it's sexy but I think he's having me on!

Actually it is very difficult writing this because as I put my head down I dribble badly and cannot control it. It is ok when I am resting with my head back. I have lost the nerves in my lower lip, as the surgeon had to cut right across the lower bone so severed the nerves. I do hope in time I will be able to control this dribbling. I have to sit up straight to control the breathing.

I am waiting for the SLT to come, as she has to give the decision if I can have my trach out today. My surgeons said "Yes" if she agrees to it. She won't be my best friend if she says "No".

I have just had the Dietician and we had fun. She was showing me how to turn off and on the feed so I can be free to go walkies. They tried to get me to flush it out and the top came off and I was covered with foul yellow food – another clean nightie! And just after a lovely Christian auxiliary nurse gave me a WONDERFUL shower and even put water on my hair!

The Physio has just been. I certainly have a whole team – like you – working with me and I am determined not to let them down. Dad took a photo of a very good-looking male Physio with me yesterday! We are building up what will be a very interesting scrapbook for when you come home.

My friend, Jo, caused a stir this morning when an enormous parcel arrived. All the nurses enjoyed opening it. It was a 'Koochie' soft toy – soft and absolutely gorgeous. Now I have to think up a name! It was such a wonderful surprise. Very impressive and the staff all enjoyed the gift with me. If you see Jo please thank her and, of course, I will when she gets back from New Zealand.

I cannot believe that this time last week I was on the operating table and really they had only just begun carving me up. What an amazing week I have been through. Please keep these letters I am writing to you, they might make interesting reading.

Going back to last evening. About 6 pm Mr Hyde (one of my surgeons) and his buddies came and found my trach tube half out. *This meant he had to make me cough violently and then I nearly broke my heart. I couldn't stop for what seemed about ½ hour and then my throat tickled and was generally irritant all evening. He told the nurse to give me a nebuliser, which didn't come until well after 10 pm when more doctors had been to see me! But as she was putting me into bed with the nebuliser, the feeding tube came off and food went everywhere!!! It was very strong smelling and awful. The nurse was not very happy! So out of bed again and another nightie. I had asked to go to bed 2 hours earlier but she just ignored and rushed about her muddled business and made matters worse. I went to bed in a muddle. Some nurses are nice and organised and seem to know what they are doing. I hope she won't be on tonight. You have to take the rough with the smooth!!! Do you remember how we used to talk about them at the National? Well, I fell asleep only to wake at 1 am, had a loo stop and gave a list to a nurse for things I needed done including plugging my CD into the mains. I fell asleep listening to a new CD JJ had brought. A lot of the CDs he gives me sound so like his voice. I'm sure he could do just as well if not better. The latest invention for JJ is to make a pill crusher. A nurse yesterday was trying to crush a pill for me with two forks!!*

Did I tell you about the auxiliary nurse with pale lavender nails with diamonds set in the middle of each nail? I asked her if they were real. She said, "I wish … I wouldn't be working here!"

I feel myself so fortunate to have had my operation. On the front page of the Telegraph there was an article saying that to meet Government targets surgeons were being forced to do non-urgent surgery, ie cosmetic etc, in front of skin cancers in Epsom Hospital.

I'll finish this later hopefully when I have had my trach out.

I love Dad bringing in all the family news so keep those e-mails coming.

I will write tomorrow what has happened this pm as Dad wants to go and get this off to you.

Lots of love to you and Lee,
Mummy

Wednesday 28th January 2004
Dearest Mary,

I am not sure how far I got yesterday, as Dad suddenly wanted to go and I had to finish it.

Anyway, Stephen came and that was nice but I do not think he is very good at stomaching hospitals! I think he was pretty amazed at my appearance! I seem to get bigger and bigger everyday. Peter also came and stayed a nice long time and told us about his weekend with Marigold (This was his new girlfriend's name and I couldn't say her real name, which was Nariko, so I called her Marigold!), the Arsenal match and then on Sunday they went to China Town, had a meal and just spent a happy time. I haven't seen Peter so relaxed and happy for a long time. Marigold works at Whitely Village and their hours clash so they don't see much of each other.

After Peter and Dad left, I had my trach out and half the staples on my neck. I now do not have my voice box anymore but have to put my fingers over my hole when I talk. I am not so clear in speech. I can hear clearly what I say but others don't. So many things to remember.

I had an awful night. First, I was meant to be connected to my feed at 10 pm but it was 11.30 pm before they did it, hence I lost that time and have to be on it longer today. Then, I was getting used to breathing on my own and wasn't breathing correctly which the SLT helped me with today. I was very hot and uncomfortable. A very long night and was not really with it when Mr Hyde and his entourage came round at 8.30 am.

The SLT came at 9.30 am and she helped me to take water, which I am getting on with. It was Blissful to have water down my throat again although it was a dreadful taste. I might ask Dad to get me some bottled water. The SLT has just come back, 1.30 pm, to see how I am getting on. She is pleased with how well I am getting the water down and is going to ask Mr Hyde if I can go on to milky drinks. She sat and talked for quite a while which I appreciated, encouraging me by saying I was doing very well especially as the op was only 8 days ago. Seems unbelievable what you can go through in just a few days.

The Dietician has been too and will alter feed. I am getting a bit of feedback at the back of my throat, which they will sort out. Won't see either the SLT or Dietician, as it is Clinic Day and they have to see the new patients like us 2 weeks ago. The SLT was telling me a bit about the radiotherapy, which will not be pleasant. Still must just get over each hurdle as it comes.

Dad will be here in a moment so will stop. Had another nice shower today which is just the best thing.

Last evening a large bouquet of 24 white tulips and supporting greenery came from Gena and Ray to my ward. They are beautiful and I think of you and your love of white tulips! I'm really tired. Oh, here is the Physio – never a moment's peace!!

I will say bye bye for now dear.
Lots of love and hugs,
Mummy

Thursday 29th January 2004

Dearest Mary,

Well, here we are again at 2.30 pm. 'Neighbours' was delayed because of the resignation of the BBC bods over the Hatton enquiry. Anyway, just managed to see a bit of it as the orthopaedic lady came to see if I had had my plaster removed. A bit fed up because it hasn't and it is meant to be done today. Still I have had my stitches out round my neck so no more sparkling clips to adorn me!

My face is still like a balloon and feels so tight and stretched. I am managing to get sips of water down and since yesterday about this time have managed a 50cc bottle and a bit more. I am longing to try something else but it is all to do with the healing of the mouth and what can be put in it. So I must be patient (Grandy's favourite word).

My lovely auxiliary nurse was back today and she and I had a good chat. There are so many nurses from all over the world to get to know, from Zimbabwe, Brazil, Jamaica, Ukraine etc!

My Dietician has just had a long talk with Dad and me about feeding at home. We are going to have a whole lot of equipment installed at home – a bit like a factory. It all sounds so complicated. Dad is coming into the hospital for 10 am on Monday to be trained by the Community Dietician – should be fun. It is the food I am worrying about more when I get home.

Just read your wonderful e-mail – what joy. You are about to embark on another holiday! Lee won't like the fishing so much in England – cold, wet and damp!! So pleased he is getting on OK in his job. Your job doesn't sound too strenuous!

I know I am apparently making excellent progress but it is incredibly difficult coping with the swallowing and speaking being still very swollen.

The team are waiting for the results of the bone analysis from the lab. The oncologist saw me today and said what is found will show them how quickly or not they have to proceed with the radiotherapy but, of course, the swelling is a problem as they cannot make my mask till that is down.

I'm looking forward to seeing the Taunton Family on Saturday but what the children will make of me I do not know.

Another long night – horrible having to sit up to feed – longing to cuddle down in my nice waterbed at home. The SLT has a waterbed back home in Australia.

Delighted about your medication. Will I recognise you when you get home? Your photos are much admired and often look at them in the night. I have showed a few nurses what I really look like!

Must go now as I am taking up visiting time with Dad. Don't want anyone other than family because it is so difficult to talk and I get hot and sweaty anyway!

Lots of love and thanks tons for your e-mail,
Mummy

Saturday 31st January 2004

Dearest Mary,

So sorry I didn't get to write you yesterday but a difficult one. Still I did have a little chat on the phone and it was lovely to hear your voice.

I'm afraid I didn't do much to make Dad's birthday happy. I had tried in the morning to get down various liquids that the SLT and Dietician gave me and was very upset when I was told in the worst scenario I might not be able to eat again through my mouth owing to the shape of my tongue and what they had done under the tongue. Apparently, I had been told all this but hadn't absorbed it. Dad was, of course, fantastic and talked with them. I had visions of never being able to travel and everything collapsing around me. They said it was early days and I suppose I get easily down when I can't do something. Still I did get down a Fruit of the Forest drink by a syringe – can you imagine your poor Mum like that?

They were short staffed yesterday and nobody was able to give me a shower and suddenly Dad arrived with me in a very food-marked nightie and also Peter and Marigold. I had wanted to look my best for Dad as it was his birthday but also to meet Marigold for the first time looking dreadful was rather sad. Still they all cheered me up. Marigold is lovely and I took to her immediately – so warm and kind.

After Peter and Marigold had left I asked Dad to shower me and it was good! Although poor Dad got wet, but it was lovely him doing it for me once again. I am so blessed to have such a very special, very wonderful husband when I think what we have been through together.

I had a quiet evening and then a nice new lady moved in opposite, up until then I had 3 men in the ward with me. After having come off my evening feed and talked to her for about ½ hour before being put on the next feed (sounds like a baby doesn't it) I had a really good night, so today I feel a lot better.

The auxiliary nurse was back on duty and took me under her wing and sat on my bed and talked to me. She is heaven sent and I wrote out the gist of what she said to me and will get Dad to send you a copy. She has also just given me a lovely shower and hair wash. I have had my trach dressing changed and the antibiotic attachment to my hand taken off.

Oh, yesterday I had all the stitches taken out of my bone graft. A real work of art and it took the nurse ages to get them out. I'm nearly ready to go home and I can hardly believe that I am at this stage so soon. I think everyone is very pleased with the progress I have made because many people just lie there – if you see what I mean. It hasn't been an easy ride but I have tried to be a good patient! I think Intensive Care will haunt me forever. Even this time last week I was struggling with a chest infection.

Gena's gorgeous tulips are now beginning not to look their best – a sure sign I should be going home!

I'm really looking forward to seeing Andrew, Liz and family this afternoon and keep trying to imagine what they are doing this morning and last night. I have enjoyed showing the photos of everyone to a few chosen people and especially what I used to look like!!!!

I hope you are having a lovely weekend. Wonderful news about your medication. It was so right for you to go away and get well. I'm glad you didn't know about me before you went away. Of course, I wish you were here but as you say having e-mail and photos makes all the difference. I am so pleased Dad got the computer all sorted out and that he got on with the digital camera when he did otherwise he wouldn't have been able to communicate with you all so easily and quickly.

I can speak quite well but not for too long as I am still very swollen and my tongue gets sore and my jaw gets sore. I also build up a lot of saliva and dribble a lot. I find it rather hard and tiring. I obviously look forward to seeing everyone but it will not be easy and will have to limit people somehow.

Well, my dear, I think this is all for now as I shall want Dad to take this with him when he comes.

It is really odd not having regular meal times. I feel really cheated. I might go and raid the refrigerator for another drink and see how I get on but it is an effort!

I wonder how dear Grandy is and what she must be thinking. It is three weeks now since I saw her.

JJ and Anne are coming on Sunday so that will be nice.

Take care of each other,

Lots of love and hugs,

Mummy

Monday 2nd February 2004

Dearest Mary,

It is 4.00 am having just woken to go to the loo. Now I can't sleep and am having a bit of a weep. Just feeling sorry for myself and wonder what the future holds. I could go on and on along those lines but I won't.

I had a lovely time with the Taunton Family on Saturday. The children were so good and absolutely gorgeous. It was hard to see them all go. They had worked hard and made me an arrangement of paper flowers in a decorated jar. They gave up their playtime when home on Friday with an Inset day to make them. It is very special.

I enjoyed JJ and Anne yesterday who were amazed at the change in me from last weekend when I couldn't even talk. We had some really good laughs and brought me a little book on – well, can't remember the name. You will have to ask them. If you are very good I might let you see it on your return. I had told Dad not to come yesterday as he has to be here by 10 am tomorrow (today now!). I wanted him to have a break.

I didn't get my shower until 12 noon yesterday having gently reminded them all morning. Apparently, showers are meant to be treats every now and again! The heat in this ward is sometimes (mostly) unbearable and I get VERY hot and sweaty. A shower is the only MUST as far as I am concerned!!

Last night, just as I thought I would be safe in my bed, they asked me to move, as someone needed my bed because it has access to all the machinery. Fortunately, I only had to move to the bed opposite but it was a nuisance because I had to try and re-organise my little bit. So we now have 3 women and 1 man.

Coping with the saliva is very difficult and I always have to have loads of tissues to hand. I know it is early days and everyone tells me how well I am doing but… I am grateful for what they have been able to do for me but…I can't pretend it is easy.

Over the weekend I have taught myself to swallow drinks and on Saturday and Sunday I had tea, Bovril, 2 milky Ensure Plus drinks so felt quite pleased with myself. I do hope in time I will be able to cope with other ordinary food. I can't imagine what it will be like if I have to be fed by PEG for the rest of my life – no wining and dining in or out and travelling not an easy option.

They have been very kind to me and in some ways I shall miss them, but I have to move on and take the next step in getting myself back into home routine, which will be lovely and, of course, being at home with my dear Alan, but it is also a bit scary without all the medical team around. Still they say that I will have all the help I need in the community.

I have to have my trach hole dressed every day and each time they take of the large plaster another layer of my skin comes off and I really dread that. My skin is quite raw. I never want a trach again – awful.

I think today is going to be quite busy with all the last minute things to be sorted out.

I have about 2 hours left of my PEG feeding. I find it difficult to work out in my mind how I will have any sort of life being tied to this PEG feeding. Still I know many live by this means but apart from feeling sorry for myself, I feel sorry for Dad. Not a happy prospect for retirement saddled with a wife with suddenly all these problems. We had so many hopes and dreams. As Andrew said when he first knew, it always happens to someone else.

Everyone here has been very encouraging and I am being positive.

You will be saying it doesn't sound like it! But most of the time with the help of everyone around, I am, but I am being honest with you when I say I have my down moments.

Just because you're not here it doesn't mean I can't let you know my feelings. If you were here I would weep with you so I've done it in letter form and am weeping as I write. I want to involve you my dear daughter not shut you out because you are not here. We have always shared so much together and so while I have been in hospital I did want to share the ups and downs.

This is a middle of the night downer and hopefully I'll put a brave face on in a few hours.

Will stop now and send loads of love hugs and kisses, Mummy

Saturday 7th February 2004

Dearest Mary,

9.00 am-ish. Hi darling. This is from a much brighter Mum, I am sure you will be pleased to know! In fact yesterday was the first day I felt more myself for ages. I have felt so poorly that I just couldn't even write a sob letter!!

1.00 pm! You think you are sitting down for a quiet moment and then everything erupts! So let's have another go!

I cannot possibly let you know all that has been going on this past week but I think Dad keeps you up to date.

This past week there has been concern for my liver. I was also coughing up lots of green phlegm, feeling sick, diarrhoea etc. I had to give samples of EVERYTHING!! These are still being tested. Blood tests until I'm sure I have no more blood to give. I had a gastro doc come and see me, then had to go for a liver scan and at the same time he did my bladder as well, I think. Also he ultrasounded my right side of face where it has been hurting and there seems to be an excess of fluid. Also more chest x-rays. You name it, I've had it!

Yesterday they had another look at my bone graft and were happy with that so then had to go down to the plaster room to have another plaster on, which goes over my elbow and nearly up to my shoulder in order to immobilise the two joints at each end of the graft. Of course, that caused a problem when I wanted my shower, as the bags we had been using were now not big enough! I asked one of the male nurses to think up something but no it needed a mere female like your mum to suggest using two bags and I showed him what to do!! I'll be running this hospital soon! I think if the bigwigs could stay a few weeks in hospital they would see what to put right and how to save money! Perhaps I could be an advisor! Actually, My Team are excellent and do not leave a leaf unturned but on the nursing side it can be frustrating to say the least.

I have now changed beds again – my 4th – and the 3rd TV that doesn't have colour. Dad is very fed up. My new bed is opposite where I was the night before my operation, by a window, which I can OPEN and at last I can sleep because it is much cooler. In the next bed is a very nice retired social worker (78), a Christian and a Tearfund supporter. We were moved in here together having been in the High Dependency ward for a week together.

Where my trach was I still have to have a dressing on it and with the continual removing of the special plastic, the skin has become raw. Today it has all come up in blisters which have to be looked at this afternoon.

On Monday the doctors want me to be taken somewhere to have a good look in my mouth. I doubt very much if I shall be out on Monday. They think that the liver problems are drug related (as Lee has already said). Join the Team Lee!

I kissed Dad on the cheek for the first time yesterday and it felt so odd. It was like giving him a half kiss because I couldn't feel my lower lip against his cheek.

I have just looked out of the window (5th floor) and seen the most beautiful rainbow.

Another break – medicines, nebuliser, Ensure Plus drink – you know the drill!

Dad will be here soon and I want to get this finished before he arrives.

Peter popped in yesterday to see me, which was lovely. Why is it that it always seems to be the time when various medics want to have a look at you?!

Saw another SLT yesterday who I also liked. Did I tell you that I have a dip in my tongue where phlegm gets caught? A nuisance. And, I suppose food will get caught too. I am doing my exercises and think a lot of you while I am doing them. Will send you a copy when I get home – I wonder when that will be?

To go back to my skin graft on my arm I noticed that it was all wrinkly and the skin they removed from my tummy had a stretch mark on it and so I now have a stretch mark on my arm! What a hoot. We have had some good laughs about that. Apparently one man had a tattoo and half of it had to be used in his mouth so now has half a tattoo on his body and half in his mouth!

I can't think of any more to say except that I am feeling a lot brighter. Oh yes, Dad and I were shown a very good book showing how the mask is made for the radiotherapy. It is quite a complex procedure. My first appointment is 23rd February – so they are not wasting any time. I am hoping I shall be through it and feeling better by my birthday – touch and go.

Sorry it has been all me so far. It is wonderful to read all your e-mails, which Dad faithfully brings in and I do thank you so very much for taking the time to write. Also thank you so much for that beautiful card – just perfect.

Do hope you had a lovely weekend away. Well done for getting off all your medication – well nearly. You must feel so much better and clearer in your head and not so lethargic. Really exciting and a wonderful answer to prayer that this year out will restore you to full health and strength once more. This is worth all the money in the world so go on enjoying your time out.

Dad has had a lot of nice meals out, which have been lovely. JJ and Anne are coming over on Sunday and they will go out for lunch again. The new restaurant in place of the motor bike shop in Shepperton is apparently very nice. Peter told me that he is going there on his birthday (about 15 of them).

I am now going to stop!
Lots of love and hugs and ½ kisses!!
Mummy

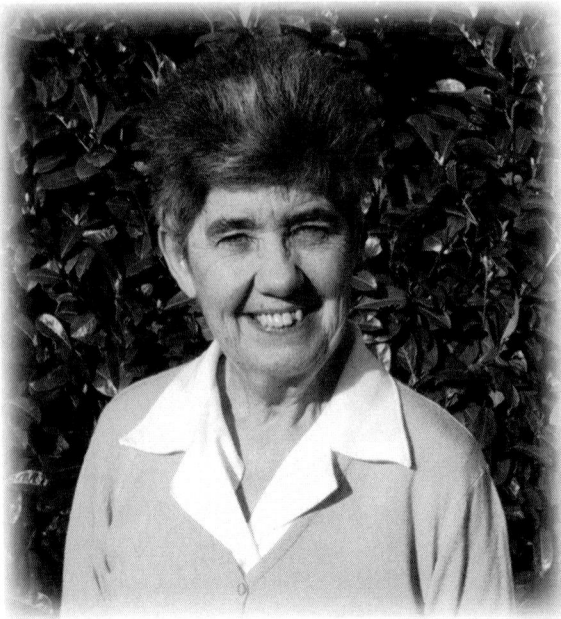
Christine before her operation

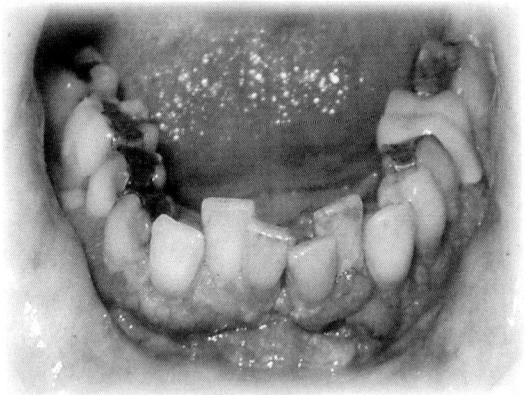
Squamous Cell Carcinoma of the oral cavity

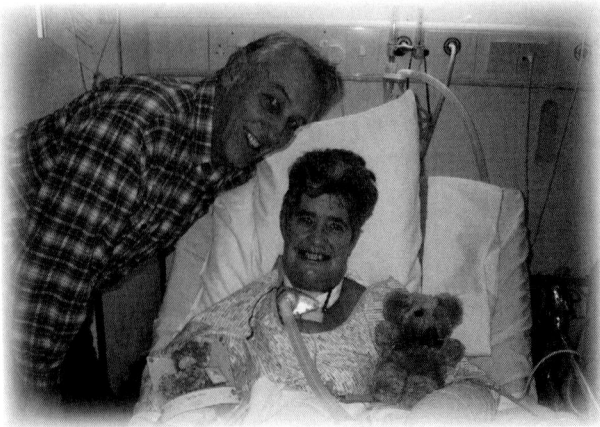
After the operation in high dependency ward

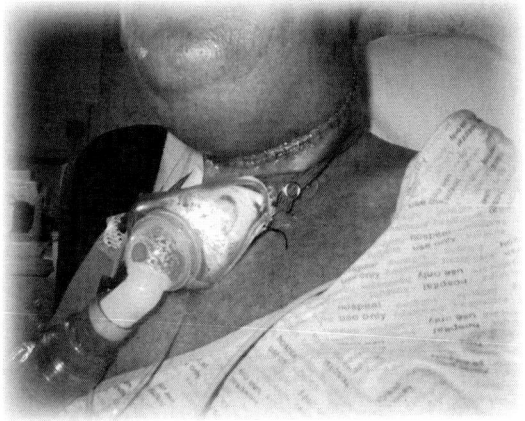

Stitching "necklace" and Tracheotomy

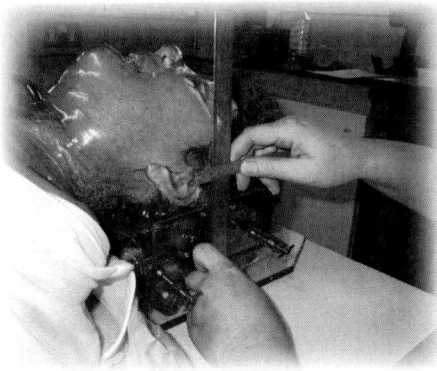

Final stages of making the mask for radiotherapy

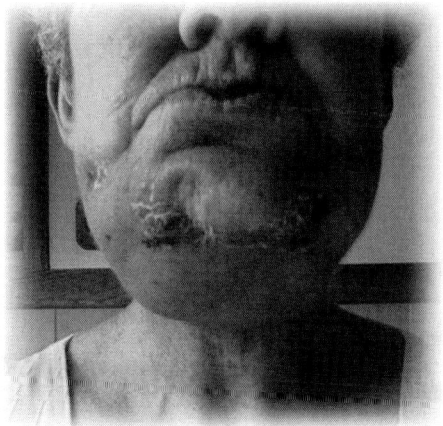

External swelling and blistering after radiotherapy

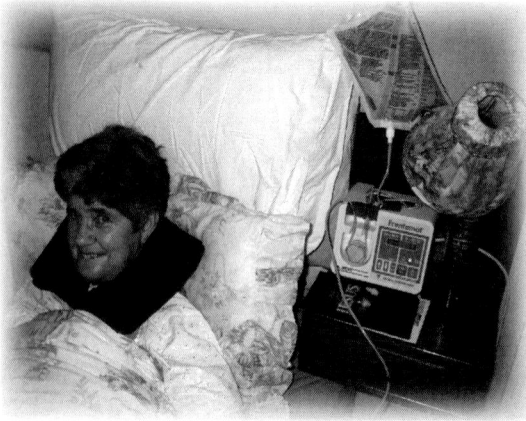

In bed at home with electronic feeding pump

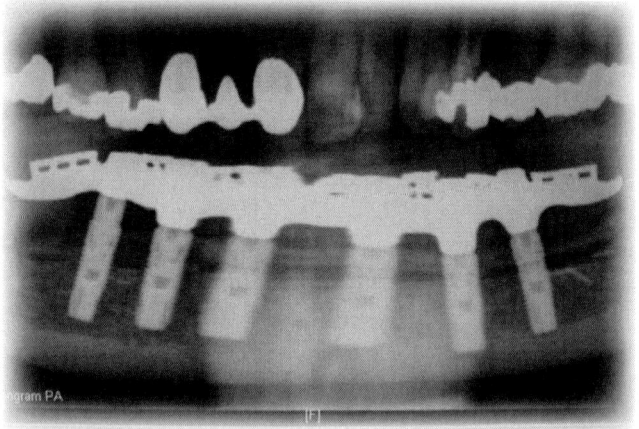

X-ray of titanium inserts for new teeth

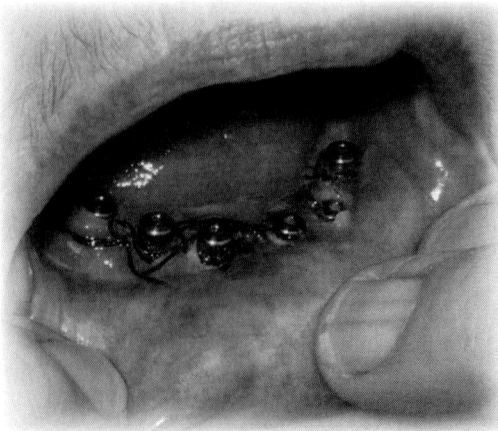

Titanium caps prior to the fitting of her new teeth

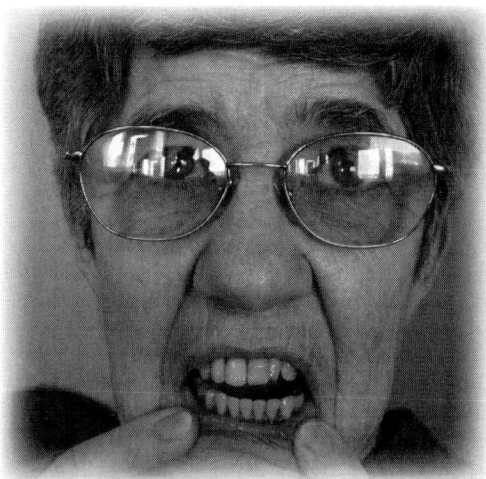
The finished job
with her new
teeth fitted

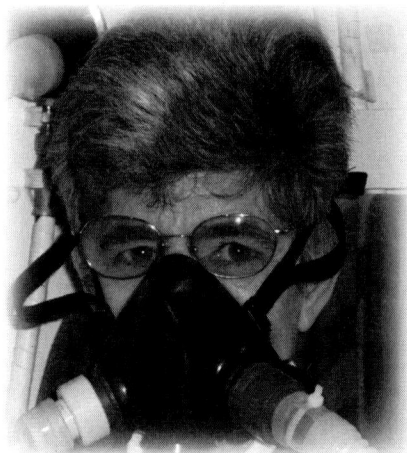
Christine in
the hyperbaric
oxygenation
chamber

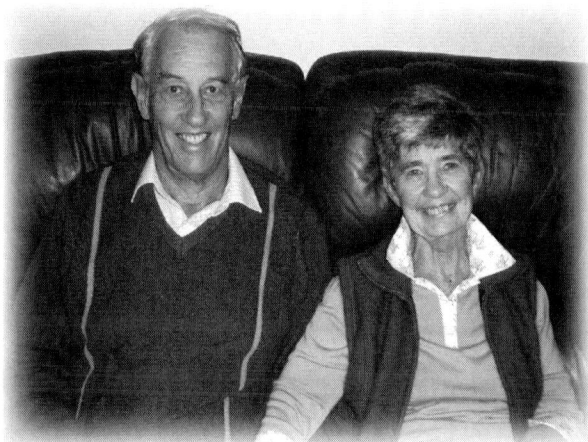
Christine
with Alan

Chapter Six
Fun with New Techniques!

*I*found it so difficult to pray during this time in hospital and friends used to say that I mustn't worry about it because they were doing the praying for me. I found this a great comfort, but the one verse that I seemed to remember and kept close to my heart was "*… underneath are the everlasting arms*", Deuteronomy Ch 33 v 27 and so I felt held by my Lord. I was given a gift of a wooden cube that had texts from the Bible all about healing. In the night when I couldn't sleep I would turn this round and round and found the words of great comfort.

When I was first told that I could try drinking some water I found that I couldn't swallow and got quite depressed thinking that I would never be able to drink or eat again. So one night when I couldn't sleep I kept trying to swallow water. How excited I was when suddenly I managed to swallow for the first time. I could hardly wait for Alan to come the next day to tell him the good news. There were many ups and downs during my hospitalisation and one day when I was down one of my doctors said I had to 'do my bit', but I didn't know what I could do to do my bit. Later a very sweet petite lady doctor sat on my bed encouraging me and talked about being positive.

Ten days after my operation it was Alan's birthday. I was really looking forward to seeing him and, of course, wanted to look my best. I had asked if I could have a shower before he came, but suddenly my SLT and Dietician were at my side wanting to see if I could get anything other than water down. This all proved absolutely disastrous and as a result I had all sorts of different liquids spilt down my nightie. I looked a mess. I was in the depths of despair and felt at rock bottom again because I thought I would never be able to get anything down but water. It was at this point that Alan appeared. This was not the way to greet one's husband on his birthday and I sobbed because I looked such a mess and was feeling very sorry for myself. Alan comforted me and tried to cheer me up and, at that point, who should come round the corner but our son, Peter. After saying "hello" he said he had someone he wanted to introduce me to and in walked Nariko. This was his girlfriend who I had never met before. She is Japanese and because I couldn't grasp her name I called her 'Marigold'! I was in despair having to greet my future daughter-in-law (although I didn't know it then) in such a dishevelled state. Peter just said, "Mum it's all right, she is a nurse so she understands". She was so sweet and although she didn't know a lot of English at that stage, I enjoyed meeting her. After Peter and 'Marigold' had gone I asked a nurse if Alan could shower me. Permission was granted and so we had a lot of fun while we coped with an arm in plaster and a tube coming out of my tummy. Alan got soaked in the process but it was well worth it and I cheered up immensely feeling fresh and clean once more before he left.

The day after this episode a lovely auxiliary nurse who was a Christian came and sat on my bed. She had a really good talk with me about trusting God and miracles. She told me about another patient who was in my ward who couldn't keep potassium in her body; it just seeped out and she had been given only three months to live. After three months she walked out alive and was still alive six months later. This was because she trusted God and not man's prediction.

So I asked God to remake my tongue and give me the joy of eating again through my mouth. He is all seeing and all knowing (not like man). I have a great God who has looked after me and I thank Him with all my heart and trust Him for the future whatever that may be. I thanked God for His servant in Dalby Ward ministering to me. Gradually I found that, with perseverance, I could manage to swallow different liquids and so I was like a baby learning new techniques!

I was due to be discharged a fortnight after my operation but this was delayed, first of all because all the support systems that I would need at home were not in place, and then I became very unwell and so more tests had to be carried out. My medical team feared a problem with my liver, so I had to have an ultrasound scan. Fortunately, nothing structural was found to be wrong and it was thought that my problems were brought about by all the post-operative medications having caused a 'blip' in the blood stream.

One of my highlights was a visit from our son, Andrew and his wife, Elizabeth, together with our three grandchildren, Emily, Annabel and Jack. They travelled up from Taunton to spend the weekend with Alan and also spent some time with me in hospital. I was a bit nervous because I wasn't sure what the children would think of their grandmother looking a bit odd. They were absolutely super and well behaved and I was very proud of them. They had made paper flowers, which they displayed in a pot and decorated; I really appreciated this, as they had given up a day off from school to make them especially for me. I had a very large cuddly cat given to me and I asked the children to give it a name. Jack suggested 'Spotty' so that was that problem solved, and Spotty was a great companion to me at that time. Elizabeth was very helpful in many ways, not least with all her wonderful letters of support and encouragement. They made the long journey from Somerset many times over the next few months, which Alan and I really appreciated and it helped to keep our spirits up.

Just before I left hospital the Macmillan nurse came to see Alan and me and explained to us the process of radiotherapy if the Consultant and Oncologist decided I needed it, which would mean the making of a mask to cover my face. After the operation, the bone that was taken away from my jaw had to be analysed in the laboratory and if there were any cancer cells left then I would have to go forward with the radiotherapy. She had a book showing how the mask was made. It all looked quite straightforward but at that time I had no idea at all what it would really mean. That I was to find out soon enough!

The great day came when I was told I could go home. This happened unexpectedly at 8.30 am when the medical team came round, and Mr Bailey said I would be better off at home than in hospital picking up any more bugs. In many ways it was a blessing in disguise that I hadn't been able to go the previous week. Although I had longed to be home, I had been very fearful about coping without all my medical support around me. Now I felt stronger and much more able to cope.

Of course, there are always lots to do before one is discharged from hospital; in my case the SLT wanted to see if I could suck down a pureed meal. I could hardly wait for lunchtime. Well, I cannot say it was the greatest meal of my life but I did manage to get most of it down so that was another landmark. I decided that it would be a good idea to keep a diary of my food intake over the next few months. This was not only for my benefit but also so the dietician would know exactly what food and how much I had managed to eat. She was then able to regulate how much liquid food she should prescribe for feeding me through my PEG. I found it very helpful in prompting me about the sort of food I could eat but it also enabled me to see how I progressed from pure liquids to more pureed/solid foods.

Alan then arrived and, after gathering all my accumulated belongings and saying a fond farewell to many of the people who had looked after me, we left after a stay of nearly a month, which was originally meant to last two weeks!

As soon as I opened the door at home, the most wonderful array of flowers greeted me! They included a beautiful bouquet

from Alan with a large sign saying, "Welcome Home Darling."
There were cards everywhere and in all I received nearly three
hundred! These were a great comfort to me and one particularly
stands out in my memory. On the front was, "God Never Said
It Would Be Easy". I have kept every single one and they occupy
three large folders.

Things didn't run altogether smoothly that first day as the
feeding pump wouldn't work. This was quite a vital piece of
equipment, as it was important that I obtained the right nutrients,
which I took in through the PEG. Fortunately, the suppliers were
able to deliver another one that day, and all was well. It took us
quite a while to get into a routine but gradually we did and Alan
proved to be an excellent nurse. He certainly should have been
awarded a special badge of recognition! Many friends wanted to
come and visit but we had to limit this because I slept so much
and was quite weak. A district nurse came regularly to check my
dressing which still covered the hole where my trach had been
and she also kept a check on my PEG hole. She took a swab
when it appeared infected but because I never heard anything
more about the results, presumed that all was well ... this was to
prove far from the case!!!

Another landmark was the removal of the plaster from my
left arm. I can see the Houseman now sawing off the plaster.
It looked most peculiar but I supposed I would get used to it!
The arm felt very weak and it was quite a while before I was
able to use it again with confidence. I felt rather self conscious
of the scar at first and, Mary, one of my friends, bought me a
long sleeve blouse for my birthday for which I was very grateful
– I don't mind now what my arm looks like! Mary would often
sneak in to see me even when there was a curfew on visiting!

Although we still hadn't received the results of the post
operative bone analysis we had to proceed with our appointments
at Charing Cross Hospital to enable the mask to be made in
case they had to go ahead with giving me radiotherapy. This

procedure was not at all pleasant, as it required lying on a solid table with my head tilted back and a mould being created, which would fit tightly over my face. This process took five visits before the mask was completed. The mask was to be placed over my face and attached to a wooden table by screws so that it was impossible for me to move. As a result of my previous back problems, this was very painful but unavoidable, and resulted on one occasion in my back going into spasm.

Then at long last we were given the results of the bone analysis. Sadly, it showed that there was a residue of cancer cells remaining at the 'margins' of the site of the operation at the back of the right mandible (near to, but below the right ear) and at the lingual margin (the floor of the mouth in front of the tongue). Naturally we were disappointed by these findings, but it was reassuring to know that the radiotherapy should eliminate these remnants.

We then had to see Dr Sarah Partridge, for her to plan my treatment. At first she was suggesting that I had four weeks (twenty sessions) at a high dose of radiation. I then asked her when I would be able to have my teeth replaced. She looked at me and said, "But you may never be able to have teeth!" On hearing this I burst into tears because I couldn't bear the thought of living the rest of my life without my bottom teeth. Having no bottom teeth caused my lower lip to fall in and I so desperately wanted to look normal again, but I also cherished the hope that I would be able to eat more normally again one day. So she left me for quite a while and when she returned said that, as my teeth meant so much to me, she would change the programme so that treatment would take place over six-and-a-half weeks (thirty-two sessions) at a reduced radiation level in the hope that it would not damage my bone so much. I was then warned of all the possible side effects which sounded horrendous but which I couldn't really take in or understand … I had no idea at that time how much suffering there would be from the radiotherapy. Dr Partridge was extremely kind and helpful overseeing the treatment that followed.

The day came for the first session of radiotherapy. I'd had various practice sessions with the staff making sure everything was just right but now it was for real. I will never forget getting onto that table, having the mask fitted and being screwed down to the table. I couldn't move, I couldn't swallow, my back hurt and I panicked. The thought of that radiation being beamed into me in a room where I was completely on my own was almost too much to bear. I was assured that if I raised my arm, the staff would then immediately come in and release me. This they had to do on a number of occasions to begin with until I got more used to it. We appealed for prayer as, at that point, I had no idea how I was going to face six-and-a-half weeks of daily treatment, and I hadn't even begun to feel the side effects. Then I managed to calm myself down and used the time while the radiation was taking place to pray for other people.

After about ten days the side effects started to 'kick in' and life really became very unpleasant. There was ulceration of my whole mouth, which was dry because of damage to the salivary glands; swelling and stiffening of the tongue making speech and swallowing more difficult; swelling, external burning and breakdown of my facial skin; all magnified by exhaustion and nausea. The only benefit of feeling so exhausted was my ability to sleep whether in bed sitting up at forty-five degrees with my food pump running for nearly eight hours during the night, sitting on the loo, and even at the bank while I was waiting to sign a document! I could be in considerable pain one moment and a few moments later, asleep. I suppose that this was one of nature's ways of protecting an individual under such circumstances.

I was given so many different medications during this period that they all had to be crushed and applied through my PEG. Alan made out a chart because it was all so complicated – what my insides were like I will never know! While my mouth was so painful I was given a cocaine mouthwash, which on one occasion was brought by courier for me from Charing Cross Hospital. It did bring relief for just a short while and I wished I could take it continually – I was warned that on no account was I to swallow it! During this period of radiotherapy at Charing Cross Hospital I quite often met up with Ray and Gena. I always hoped that our appointments might coincide and when they did we were able to swap notes and try to encourage one another. We both found it so hard and, as time went on, increasingly difficult to talk. Gena and Alan were always there trying to keep our spirits up and attending to our every need.

While I was undergoing treatment at Charing Cross hospital, I was continually being monitored with blood tests and a care team comprising a speech therapist, dietician, oral hygienist and Macmillan nurse. All the staff in the department were very supportive and nothing was too much trouble. I did have to have a blood transfusion at one point, as there was a deficiency of haemoglobin. I was encouraged to keep up my tongue and mouth exercises even though my mouth was so painful.

Towards the end of the treatment I was warned that the side effects could get worse even after the radiotherapy had finished, as the effects of the therapy continue in just the same way as food continues cooking in a microwave oven even after it has been turned off! Looking back now I have no idea at all how I survived that period. I was so fortunate to have so many prayerful people surrounding me, also a super team of radiotherapists who were very kind and encouraging.

We arrived home having made our last journey for the radiation treatment on the 23rd April to find on our doorstep a lovely bouquet of flowers from Gena and Ray to cheer me up. This meant so much to us and brought tears to my eyes knowing how much they were suffering too. I was glad that I had finished radiotherapy by my birthday at the beginning of May because my brother, David and his wife, Rowena, were due to be in England for a short visit enabling them to see our mother. I hadn't seen my mother since just before my operation so it was a special way of celebrating my birthday to be able to see them. David brought my mother from her residential home and I prepared a simple birthday tea which, of course, I couldn't eat! It was lovely to see them but they didn't stay long because I tired very easily.

I began to be able to have visitors and I enjoyed sitting in the garden, as we happened to be having a lovely spell of sunshine. Alan bought me three floppy sun hats (blue, pink and cream) to wear in the garden as I had been warned never to let my face get burnt. I remember my friend, Pam, kept me on my toes regarding my tongue exercises and kept getting me to stick my tongue out and see how far it would go whenever we met. We corresponded by e-mail regularly and she often made me laugh. Mavis came to see me often, and once after spending a while with me in the garden, went home and wrote me a lovely poem. She was often just given poems, which she wrote down and sent by e-mail to me, like this one:

My True Friend

When we were young how good it was
To pass the time with fun and joy
It mattered not who were our friends
They all were counted – girl and boy

This worked for years whilst then in school
But time it changed once more
For as we grew and wise became
True friends we'd have in store

We'd have that special little chat
We'd share our deepest fear
It was but with a handful
Those now we'd hold so dear

For life was not to be all flowers
Of lovely things to share
We'd have our times of broken hearts
And moments of despair

We'd hit the harbour wall at times
We'd battle with the storm
But still our friends would all be there
When life was not the norm

But now the storms are really fierce
The stops are fully out
We're stretched beyond our wildest dreams
We really must not doubt.

For all those friends who watch with you
A greater Friend have they
He is the One – the greatest Friend
Who'll see you through each day

He is the greatest Friend of all
He'll never let you go
Unlike us feeble human friends
True love to you He'll show

I thank the Lord for all our friends
They've been with me for years
They've ridden with me through the dark
And wiped away my tears

But still much greater than all that
Is Him the Greatest Friend
He'll see you through this awful time
With Him there is no end

Our human friends can make a pie
Or maybe make a cake
But this great Friend can give the peace
A difference this will make

Just peace and joy when all else fails
And guidance He will send
So please just hang on through this storm
With Him, your Greatest Friend.

Mavis Duncan 26.3.04

Colin came one afternoon to play classical music and spiritual songs on his guitar, and his wife, Di, read to me. In fact, over the next few months, I had so many visits from friends near and far that I cannot name them all. I just want to say how much they meant to me that they put themselves out and often made long journeys to be with me for only a short while. This helped to keep my spirits up, and was a great encouragement and all part of my healing process.

Sandra, our Pastoral Assistant at church, came and saw me and suggested that she organise someone to co-ordinate the meals that friends wanted to bring us so that we didn't get ten cottage pies all at one go! She also wrote Alan an e-mail showing how important it was for him to be looked after both practically and emotionally and I was very grateful for the loving care he was given.

After I had finished my radiotherapy I was given an appointment to see Mr Bailey at Kingston Hospital and while we were waiting our turn, we started talking to a lady who had undergone an operation for mouth cancer in St George's a couple of months before mine. We struck up a friendship with Maureen and her husband Ron and often found ourselves waiting side by side to see the same Consultant. We found that they lived quite near us and so we were able to visit each other in our homes and were often on the telephone when either of us needed to chat something through. It was so helpful to be able to compare notes and encourage one another.

I was looking forward to seeing Mr Bailey, as I was wondering how I would ever get through this dreadful time. I was feeling very down but in spite of all my problems he was very pleased with my progress. He said it was normal that I was feeling low because he had anticipated that there would be highs and lows. Then without saying any more he made the sign of the cross on my forehead with his thumb and put a hand on my head. This meant so much and really encouraged me.

Little by little I began to regain my strength and started looking forward to our holiday in Cornwall at the beginning of July. But there was another hurdle to overcome before I could get there. This hurdle was the removal of my PEG. Of course, I wanted it removed; it was a great inconvenience although the amount of food I took through it was being slowly reduced as I managed to suck down soft food and purees – I spent many hours making soup and juicing fruit and vegetables of all kinds. But I also knew that once it was removed I would be wholly responsible for feeding myself. I was very fearful and did not feel at all confident that I could do this.

An appointment was made at Kingston Hospital to see a nurse who specialised in removing PEGs. I arrived feeling very unsure still but this nurse talked to me for about an hour and really understood how I was feeling. It was like a bereavement having the PEG taken out, as I had been dependent on it for so long to keep me alive. It only took moments for her to remove it, however, and the hole healed up in no time at all. So now I was on my own and I started to make preparations for travelling, which involved, amongst other things, making enough home-made soup to last the two weeks we would be away. It all seemed so unreal that I was actually well enough to make the journey to Cornwall. I felt like a child being let out to play again.

Chapter Seven
A Roller Coaster Ride

We had one week's holiday on the Roseland Peninsula in Cornwall followed by a further week at a friend's cottage in Winkleigh in Devon. The weather was not very kind to us and I think we managed to sit on the beach once! It certainly wasn't warm enough for any sea bathing but we were able to swim in an indoor pool during the first week. The main thing was that we were able to enjoy God's beautiful creation away from all the strains and stresses of the past few months. Whilst in the West Country we visited some of our friends, and one family we visited will always stand out in my memory. When we had shared what I had been through, they asked whether they could pray for me. Sam their eldest son who at the time was only eight said the most beautiful prayer for my healing without any help from his parents. This really touched me.

While we were coping with my cancer, friends suggested that we should have various projects or goals to work towards which we thought was a very good idea. One of these projects was to redesign our bathroom, which helped to divert our minds away from my cancer. We arranged for it to be gutted while we were away because I didn't want to cope with all the dust while living at home. So it was a real uplift to come back to find the bathroom well on the way to completion.

We were very thankful when in July Tearfund kindly allowed Alan to go onto a three-day week for the remaining six months before his retirement to enable him to spend as much time with me as possible and to help me with my recovery. This was actually an employees' option in line with the charity's policy relating to the final six months before retirement age, but it was not always possible to arrange this for staff. Many of Alan's colleagues were amazed at the way he handled my illness and said that the way his strong faith and trust in God shone through in his life had increased their faith as well.

On our return from holiday we went for our last visit to Kingston Hospital before being transferred back to my local hospital in Ashford. Mr Bailey was delighted with the progress of the healing process of my mouth even though my tongue was still swollen on one side and I experienced a burning sensation when eating some foods and using my mouthwash. I was told that this would probably go on for another six months but sadly to this day I still experience an extremely sore tongue. The SLT and Dietician were both satisfied with how I had persevered with my exercises and my attempts to vary my diet. My one disappointment, however, was that Mr Creedon would not be able to consider fitting new teeth for at least another six months – if at all. I was encouraged to be patient, as the mouth had to be completely healed before the next step could be considered.

I was then told I would be seen monthly for a check up and I found it very reassuring that my medical team were going to keep an eye on me and not leave me in a state of limbo. It was lovely to be back under the care of my local hospital at last and I was given a warm welcome by the team there. It was great to see Linda, the receptionist in the Oral Department who had made my appointments over so many years. She is always so helpful and cheerful and I am never afraid to telephone her when I need a bit of help or advice from either Mr Bailey or Mr Creedon.

I realised that I just had to get on with my life the best I could, and that I was extremely fortunate to be alive and reasonably well again. One of the very difficult things I had to come to terms with was not being able to eat out socially. It suddenly came home to me in a big way that, whenever an event is held, it almost always includes food of some kind. It is very hard to have to ignore the gorgeous food that had often been prepared. I was helped greatly with this problem when I talked with a friend three years later who suffered from Coeliac disease. She also found it difficult to eat out not knowing exactly what was in the food. She said that she didn't look at the food but at the people and as I have always enjoyed getting alongside people I knew that this was the way forward for me.

I certainly had many down periods and during one of these times I developed a real fear of death. On 20th August 2004 I met with the Lord very early one morning and He spoke to me in an amazing way through Psalm 91 v 1: "… *He who dwells in the shelter of the Most High will rest in the shadow of the Almighty.*" I felt He was saying to me that if I belong to Him I have nothing to fear. He gave me excitement about meeting all the saints who had gone on before. I just thanked my Lord for this assurance and revelation.

There was another time when I felt ugly and useless but again the Lord spoke to me while I was reading a chapter called God's Power in Your Weakness in Rick Warren's book, *The Purpose Driven Life*. It reminded me how the Bible is full of the amazing achievements of imperfect and unremarkable people whom God has used despite their weaknesses. He has to use flawed people – they are the only sort He has to choose from. I was greatly encouraged when I read in the Bible "*I am with you; that is all you need. My power shows up best in weak people*". 2 Corinthians Ch 12 v 9a (LB) Ever since this time people have said to me "You should write your cancer story", but it is only now, just over three years since my dreadful ordeal, that I have been able to do so, and only then after a continual nagging in my innermost being. I can only conclude that God wants me to write this story as a testimony to His love and care for me, and as an encouragement to others who may be going through similar experiences.

As 2004 progressed towards September I got very excited

because Mary and Lee were due home from their year away travelling the world. We made sure we were at the airport in plenty of time to watch them coming down the Arrival passage. What sheer joy I felt that they were home and we thanked and praised Almighty God for keeping them safe and well during their time away. Mary told me later that when she had said goodbye to me she had this feeling that when she next saw me I would be looking different. At the time of her departure we had no idea of what was going to happen to me.

Our friends Mavis and Bruce said that as soon as I felt well enough, they wanted to take us for a day out in their camper van. One lovely sunny day in October we boarded their van and were taken to the New Forest, a place I hadn't been to since Alan and I had celebrated our Silver Wedding Anniversary there. After touring around for a while Bruce found a lovely quiet spot where ponies enjoyed grazing, to have our lunch. Mavis had prepared a lovely and appropriate meal, which I was able to enjoy and then we played Scrabble and Tri-ominos. The time passed all too quickly and it seemed in no time at all we were back home having had a very special day out.

In August 2004 Alan and I decided that we would like to go away somewhere to be able to spend time with God seeking His healing for me and guidance for the future, as Alan would be retiring at the end of the year. After being recommended to a place in Dorset called Green Pastures, a Christian Centre of Pastoral Care and Healing, we booked in for a weekend in October. The weekend was very special but it also brought home to me how weak I was. Tears kept falling as I kept reliving many aspects of what I had gone through during the previous months. The Head of the centre suggested that it would be a good idea if I had some counselling when I returned home.

It was Gena who told me about The Mulberry Centre (West London's Cancer Support and Information Centre) which is an independent charity housed in its own building on the site of the West Middlesex Hospital. Alan and I decided that we would visit this Centre and see if I could get some counselling there. We found that they did all sorts of different activities for cancer sufferers and their partners; I opted for some counselling and massage, and I was also encouraged to join a support group that met once a week.

Maureen also agreed to join the group, which I found helpful because we had both had mouth cancer while the others in the group had experienced many other different cancers. Fortunately, Maureen hadn't had to have radiotherapy but she was also looking forward to having some new teeth. In the end she only had her teeth a couple of weeks before I had mine. We used to compare notes over the phone every time we had been to see our Consultant! I felt this was all part of my journey along the road to gaining complete healing. I found all these different sessions helpful not least being able to listen and share our different experiences. The staff was so kind and caring and the whole place created an atmosphere of peace.

I was forever asking my consultants when I would be able to start the process of implants for my teeth. It certainly was an endurance of patience because I had to wait until they were absolutely sure that the bone in my jaw was strong enough to support the implants, and it was not until a whole year later in February 2005 that I was told that I could proceed to the next stage. I attended a pre-operation appointment when it was explained to me in detail the process by which my teeth were to be fitted, including computerised photographs of the various steps. The Specialist undertaking this procedure was Mr Creedon. I was booked to go into Ashford Hospital on February 23rd, subject to the availability of a bed. Imagine our surprise and shock when the bed manager phoned us in the afternoon of the actual day to say that I couldn't come into hospital because I had the MRSA bug. Alan and I were absolutely stunned because this was the first we had ever heard about it. A phone call to our doctor confirmed that my Health Centre had been informed the previous March by the Laboratory at St Peters Hospital but neither Mr Creedon nor I had been told. I was heartbroken, frustrated and angry that I hadn't been told the previous year when the swab of my PEG hole had been taken. I could have been treated then and possibly not have suffered so much during my radiotherapy. I had also developed eczema on my legs, which caused me a great deal of discomfort. When I was swabbed it was found that I had the bug in my eczema and as soon I had got rid of the bug, my legs became eczema free!

Alan was found to have MRSA as well as a result of his caring for me and having to clean my various dressings. Therefore, we both had to go through a very strict regime to rid our bodies of this miserable bug before I could be admitted into hospital. This entailed taking antibiotics by mouth and a mouthwash and a spray into our noses. We had to shower and wash our hair every day with a pink solution, and all our clothes, bed linen and towels had to be washed every day too. At the end of a week we had to report to the hospital for swabs to be taken, after which we had to wait about another week for the results. We were not deemed free of the bug until we had had three clear swabs at weekly intervals. What joy it was when the final result came through indicating that we were both bug-free. Of course, Mr Creedon was very frustrated because he lost a whole morning's surgery time and my nurse had spent quite a long time laying out all the instruments. Only when I had the all clear, was Mr Creedon able to arrange a date for my admittance into hospital, which of course meant a further delay.

We were very excited when at last we were given 11th May 2005 as the date but of course we had to secure a bed first! The great day dawned but to our frustration there were no beds available; we were told to telephone early the next morning at 7.30 am. Again no beds were available. Then finally, at 8.30 am we were told to come in right away and I was down in theatre at ten thirty not returning to the ward until three in the afternoon. Alan said I looked like a gerbil with the swelling, but Mr Creedon was very pleased with the way the operation had gone. He had been able to remove the three titanium ties that had been put in to bind the bone taken from my arm to the remaining jawbone at the time of the original operation. He then drilled and inserted six titanium screws into the lower jaw as the foundation for the new teeth. After spending a night in hospital, I was discharged with a regime of medication to be taken over the next two weeks involving twenty-three 'actions' every day! We were also encouraged by the surgeon's report that, after a thorough inspection of my mouth, tongue and throat, he could find no sign of any further growths despite the soreness I continued to feel. He put this discomfort down to the continuing after-effects of the radiotherapy. I then had to wait for another six months before the next phase of the treatment could be commenced in case the titanium screws were rejected.

Whilst in Torquay for our church's house party in October of that year, we visited Cockington Forge. We found a Calligrapher there whom we asked to copy our special verse (Proverbs 3 v 5–6) that was on the mirror in our bedroom. We were absolutely thrilled when the finished product arrived in the post; it was just what we wanted. It is now hanging over our mirror and greets us as we wake up every morning.

I patiently waited another six months, but never let Mr Creedon forget when the six-month period would be up! I then had my jaw x-rayed to see what condition the implants were in, and was very relieved when Mr Creedon said that all was well and that we could proceed to the next stage. Everything that happened to me over that period was a milestone and I got more and more excited when I was able to start another procedure. So at the beginning of December I commenced the first of seven fortnightly visits to the hospital which would cover the next three months. It was decided that I should be treated as an outpatient (to avoid any further problems with MRSA). The first session involved cutting open the flap which covered the implants, removing plugs from inside the implants, replacing them with screw-in caps to enable easy access for the following sessions and then stitching the flap up again leaving the screw caps exposed! As I watched the various procedures over the next few months, it was like watching a little boy playing with his Meccano – so many minute screws and caps which had to be fitted together. I had several sessions taking mouldings and measurements and preparing a dummy bridge. Also different caps had to be fitted to the implants for securing the final bridge.

In anticipation of my final appointment to have my longed-for teeth fitted, and towards which everyone had worked so hard for me, I decided it would be a nice to make my wonderful team a cake. I iced it and made two sprays of pink spring blossoms out of petal paste with ribbons attached. I asked Erica, a sugarcraft acquaintance of mine, if she would be kind enough to make me a bottom row of teeth out of petal paste, and she was delighted to have a go at this unusual request. I then finished the cake off with the words "Thank you with a smile".

On the 29th March I woke at 7.39 am and wrote down: "This is the day I get my teeth!" Such a longed-for day! Two years ago I was told that I might never have my bottom teeth. God directed me to Psalms 91 v 14–16.

"Because he loves Me," says the Lord,
"I will rescue him;
I will protect him for he
Acknowledges My Name.
He will call upon Me, and I will answer him
I will be with him in trouble,
I will deliver him and honour him.
With long life will I satisfy him
And show him My salvation."

Thank You Father that You have answered our prayers. I weep with joy that You have given me life to enjoy with my Alan, family and friends. Thank You for each and every one of them.

So it was with great excitement that I arrived for my appointment armed with a big white box containing my cake! I was finally fitted with a 'bridge' made of gold with twelve acrylic teeth – two more than originally anticipated! It was amazing to see Mr Creedon finally securing the bridge to the six implants, even using a miniature wrench set at a specific 'torque' setting as if he was fitting sparking plugs to the engine of a car! I was given a mirror to view the final effect and was amazed that my face immediately looked almost back to how it was before my surgery. It was explained to me the importance of cleaning each of the six holes created by the bridge after EVERY meal to avoid infection. Again another learning process for me as it was very difficult cleaning from inside the mouth through the holes with a special brush.

I then presented my cake and there were smiles all round. I don't know who claimed the sugar teeth! Alan took some photos of me with some of my team who had been so caring and encouraging to me over such a long period of time and I am extremely grateful to each and everyone who had a part in my recovery. It was a very joyous occasion. Mr Creedon was very pleased with the way everything fitted although he explained that it would be some time before the inside of my mouth and particularly my tongue moulded into their new shape to accommodate the teeth. This immediately became apparent as, despite the teeth feeling very comfortable, I found that I was biting my tongue, the insides of my cheeks and bottom lip. Worse, however, was to follow. Although I had been warned that eating and perhaps speaking might be difficult, eating in fact proved quite painful. Owing to the fact that I had no saliva and my tongue had a limited range of movement, even swallowing the same type of food that I had been eating for the last two years proved troublesome, let alone trying anything a little more solid. I found chewing quite impossible with my tongue continuing to be very sore and stinging continually. I had longed to have some toast and marmalade and thought that once I had my teeth all would be well. How wrong I was, and I experienced a great disappointment. From the excitement of getting my new teeth and hoping to be 'normal' once more, I lapsed into despair, which I would have to come to terms with.

Just after I had had my teeth fitted, a very old family friend in Edinburgh who had retired from being a physiotherapist, knowing that my mouth was still feeling so miserable after the radiotherapy, told me about Hyperbaric Oxygenation. This is a treatment where Multiple Sclerosis sufferers gain help from breathing in pure oxygen through a mask while in a pressure tank. (Divers undergo this treatment to recover from the bends). The idea was that if I was able to breathe in pure oxygen this would expedite the healing of my tongue. We decided to proceed with this treatment having got the consent of Mr Bailey.

The nearest place where I would be able to receive this treatment was at the Harrow MS Therapy Centre, so Alan and I travelled there to look round and to meet the Manager, Lynn. She explained to us exactly what would be involved and I tried on a mask and sat in the chamber just to familiarise myself with everything before I went for my first treatment. Lynn told me that the whole session would last about one-and-a-half hours. Fifteen minutes to dive down to thirty-three feet, one hour sitting breathing deeply at that level, and then another fifteen minutes coming up. This would be excellent reading time! Lynn and her team showed me a great deal of kindness and it was always a joy to be with them.

My tongue was a constant misery so anything that might give me any hope at all we felt was worth proceeding with. I also tried many different gels, mouthwashes and sprays to give me artificial saliva but they all irritated my tongue. I was sure that there must be a painkiller that would take the pain away from my tongue but sadly there is nothing. Perhaps one day a painkiller will be made specifically for mouth problems. Before I lost my saliva I had no idea of what an important function it performs in the mouth. It helps to break down and digest food, helps with speech and also acts as a protective film for the teeth. Therefore without saliva I was told to brush my own teeth with a fluoride gel every day which will help to protect them from decay.

I started my treatment at the beginning of May 2006 when I travelled to the MS Centre in Harrow five days a week for four weeks, after which I reduced this treatment to twice a week for the next three months. I felt I did see some improvement to the side of my tongue but it was still very uncomfortable. I then had a break while we travelled overseas but decided to have another go in July and August 2007, which again involved travelling to Harrow twice a week. This time I didn't think this treatment helped to reduce the pain any further, so I decided not to continue with it any more.

Just before I started on this treatment our friends Alan and Lesley in New Zealand sent me a handkerchief which they had prayed over in accordance with the scripture: "... *so that even handkerchiefs and aprons that had touched him were taken to the sick, and their illnesses were cured ...*" Acts Ch 19 v 12. Living on the other side of the world, of course, had prevented them from praying over me personally, so when I received the handkerchief from them I was very moved and it now has a special place in my Bible.

In July 2006 I had one of my check ups with Mr Bailey and Alan said that he was praying for a miracle that my saliva would return but Mr Bailey said, "It will be a miracle when you accept your condition". I went away and thought a great deal about this comment.

Alan and I follow the Bible reading notes *Every Day with Jesus* written by the late Selwyn Hughes and on 17th October

2006 he was commenting on the verse: "*And we know that in all things God works for the good of those who love Him.*" Romans Ch 8 v 28. The commentary went on to say: "*Some of the events which affect us may, in themselves, be evil, but God works in and through those events to turn them to good. The things that happen do not necessarily have a purpose; a purpose has to be given to them.*"

I underlined these words and wrote by the side of them, "*My book?*" The previous day Selwyn had commented on the verse: "*This will result in your being witnesses to them,*" Luke Ch 21 v 13 saying: "*Everything is an opportunity for those who follow Christ – providing they know how to adjust their sails so that they are driven in the right direction. 'All winds blow us towards God's goal, but the soul has to be set in the right position'. When we are aware of this secret then we can face every situation with the conviction that a blessing can be derived from it.*"

This I thought would help me to accept my situation and use it in the best possible way, and so when I saw Mr Bailey after Christmas I was able to share that with him. However, it was at this point that I was given another ray of hope concerning the pain I was experiencing with my tongue when Alan got in touch with my Oncologist, Dr Sarah Partridge at Charing Cross Hospital. I still hadn't got permission to use her name in my book as she had been on Maternity leave, so in October Alan tried once more to phone her to see if she was back. She had returned only that week, gladly gave permission and then asked how I was. Alan explained to her about my very sore tongue. She then asked if we had ever thought about trying Clinical Hypnotherapy, explaining that this is used as part of pain management. She left us to think it over and let her know if we were interested in this treatment.

As we had only heard about the 'stage type' of hypnosis we were rather dubious, but Dr Partridge assured us that it was nothing like that, so we did our own research. We understood that a person will not do anything under clinical hypnotherapy that is against his or her will. This form of treatment is about enabling the patient to gain greater control of the mind – that is, empowering rather than taking control away.

Having been assured that it was a good therapy and also had the blessing of my consultant, Mr Bailey, we decided to take up Dr Partridge's offer; she was also a trained hypnotherapist so we were very happy to proceed under her care.

At my first appointment Dr Partridge explained very clearly what would happen, that I was in complete control and could get off the bed at any time I wanted to. I likened it to very deep relaxation and in that mode, Dr Partridge talked to my subconscious. She also taught me how to put myself into a deep state of relaxation so that I could continue to derive benefit in the future. I had five one-hour sessions which I found extremely helpful and I was feeling far more positive about the future. I could now manage without my saliva gel and other medication that had helped give me saliva but irritated my tongue so much that it was becoming unbearable. I felt much more in control of my mouth, and I was also given permission not to try to eat fruit which, being acidic, was another great source of irritation. We keep being told to have so much fruit each day so it was a relief to be told that I didn't have to! Actually, I like fruit and feel sad that it causes me such a problem, but Dr Partridge suggested that during my relaxed state I could imagine myself eating fruit and in this way satisfy my desire for it. One part of this process is imagery, trying to imagine enjoying things I now cannot do.

Although I said that I thought I had been able to accept my situation, Dr Partridge identified that I hadn't grieved for my loss and she helped me to do just that. At the end of the session I found myself crying which was a tremendous release.

I found this therapy very beneficial and, although I am not out of pain, it has helped me to be positive and cope better with my condition.

Conclusion

Owing to the delay in getting my teeth we had had to postpone our planned trip to Canada and also New Zealand and Australia. Now that I had my teeth we decided to try and organise these trips even though eating wasn't going to be as easy as we had hoped. My mother had always longed for the time I would go and see my brother, David and his wife Rowena, in Canada and then come back and tell her all about it. Sadly, she died in November 2004 soon after my operation so I was never able to have the joy of telling her about my trip; nevertheless, I still wanted to go to Canada and see where David had settled in his retirement. In September 2006 we ventured forth and spent three weeks touring, starting in Vancouver and then travelling on the Rocky Mountaineer to Banff and then on to Toronto taking in the Niagara Falls before spending a week with David and Rowena in Wellington, Ontario. We finished our tour by staying four days in New York before flying home. I took with me some protein drinks, which were most useful on the aeroplanes when it was impossible to get food that I could eat.

Actually, my diet is very simple! Every main meal must have mashed potatoes, very soft vegetables and plenty of gravy. Meat is cut up very small and mixed up with the potatoes, vegetables and gravy. Plain white fish and mashed potatoes with parsley sauce would make another meal. Any sort of milk pudding but not chocolate. The acid in fruit and tomatoes makes my tongue sting unbearably, so that's another 'no-go' area. I have bananas and plain yoghurt most days, and plenty of homemade soups in which I soak a piece of wholemeal bread. I cannot eat anything that is dry, ie cakes, pastry, bread etc.

Having accomplished this amazing trip, it gave me courage to plan our longed-for holiday to New Zealand and Australia. We had met Alan and Lesley on a trip to the Holy Land about twelve years before and they had asked us to go and visit them one day. We promised we would when Alan retired, but, of course, we had no idea that this would have to be postponed somewhat. Alan said he would help us plan our time in New Zealand because for the first seventeen days before we met up with them, we decided to tour South Island in a camper van. We then flew to North Island and were met by our friends and enjoyed an unforgettable week with them and great Christian fellowship. One of their sons kindly put us up for a couple of nights while we were in Wellington and then we drove to Alan and Lesley's home in Wanganui. After spending two days there we drove to Rotorua and spent four days in their brother-in-law's beautiful holiday home by Lake Rotoiti.

We shared with them about the book I hoped to write one day and we had lots of fun trying to think up a title!

We also had friends in Australia, Norman and Mavis, who we had got to know when they visited our church, All Saints, Laleham, Middx in 2003, and had invited us to come and stay. Before we joined them in Rockhampton we spent a week in Sydney staying with Joyce who was an old friend of Norman's. She became a firm friend and has since visited us in our home in England.

We had a wonderful time with Norman and Mavis who arranged for us to go on a trip to the Barrier Reef in their brother-in-law's fishing boat for three days. Before my operation I had always enjoyed snorkelling but without my teeth I hadn't been able to hold a snorkel in place, so now, armed with my teeth, I really wanted to have a go. I did just about manage to hold the snorkel in my mouth but, oh how the salt water stung my tongue and mouth! I persevered and saw the amazing coral colours on the reef and many wonderful fish, it was worth it but it was also at a cost; my mouth stung even more for days to come. We then spent three days on Frazer Island where we enjoyed walking in the rain forest, and tramped over sand dunes to a lake where we bathed and drove along an eighty-mile beach. After this we toured in Mavis and Norman's luxury camper van until sadly we had to leave them at Brisbane and fly to Cairns for our final week in Australia. On the way home we stopped off in Hong Kong where we visited one of Alan's ex colleagues at Tearfund and then on to Bangkok where I was able to see for myself the awful poverty endured by so many. Alan had visited Bangkok when he had worked for Tearcraft and Tearfund and therefore was able to show me where he had been many years before. I felt extremely blessed that I had been able to experience so much in such a short while.

As I reflect on my journey it has been a roller coaster ride; being supported in many ways and lifted out of the valley, only to return when some new problem occurred, thus showing the value of ongoing prayer and practical support from family and friends. Going through my personal dark tunnel, I realised how much I had taken for granted in the past. I had no idea what an important part my mouth, tongue, teeth and saliva played in my everyday life – we certainly don't know how valuable something is until we lose it – but for every shadow there is a light and I know that, though God was with me in the valley, He never lets anyone stay there. He has brought me out into the light to be His witness in the world and to be able to continue to enjoy my family and watch my grandchildren grow up. For this I shall be eternally grateful. None of us know what each day will bring, but I am glad that Jesus has been my Saviour for many years and, even though my life has been rocky at times, He gives Alan and me a peace that passes all understanding, and we know that He will be with us until He calls us home.

Father, I place into your hands
The things I cannot do.
Father, I place into Your hands
The things that I've been through.
Father, I place into Your hands
The way that I should go,
For I know I always can trust You.

Copyright © *Thankyou Music* 1975.

ISBN 142517080-3

9 781425 170806